W9-BXE-501

Withdrawn

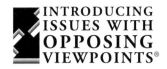

INTRODUCING
ISSUES WITH
OPPOSING
VIEWPOINTS®

Animal Rights

Other books in the Introducing Issues
with Opposing Viewpoints series:

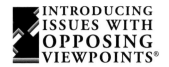
**INTRODUCING
ISSUES WITH
OPPOSING
VIEWPOINTS®**

Animal Rights

William Dudley, *Book Editor*

Bonnie Szumski, *Publisher, Series Editor*
Helen Cothran, *Managing Editor*

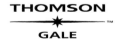
GREENHAVEN PRESS
An imprint of Thomson Gale, a part of The Thomson Corporation

THOMSON
™
GALE

Detroit • New York • San Francisco • San Diego • New Haven, Conn. • Waterville, Maine • London • Munich

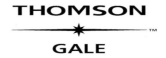

THOMSON
™
GALE

LIBRARY OF CONGRESS CATALOGING-IN-PUBLICATION DATA

Animal rights / William Dudley, book editor.
    p. cm. — (Introducing issues with opposing viewpoints)
Including bibliographical references and index.
    ISBN 0-7377-3457-4 (lib. : alk. paper)
    1. Animal rights. I. Dudley, William, 1964– II. Series.
    HV4708.A5492 2006
    179'.3—dc22
 	
                                                                    2005055133

Printed in the United States of America

Contents

Chapter 3: Are Scientific Experiments on Animals Justified?

Foreword

I ndulging in a wide spectrum of ideas, beliefs, and perspectives is a critical cornerstone of democracy. After all, it is often debates over differences of opinion, such as whether to legalize abortion, how to treat prisoners, or when to enact the death penalty, that shape our society and drive it forward. Such diversity of thought is frequently regarded as the hallmark of a healthy and civilized culture. As the Reverend Clifford Schutjer of the First Congregational Church in Mansfield, Ohio, declared in a 2001 sermon, "Surrounding oneself with only like-minded people, restricting what we listen to or read only to what we find agreeable is irresponsible. Refusing to entertain doubts once we make up our minds is a subtle but deadly form of arrogance." With this advice in mind, Introducing Issues with Opposing Viewpoints books aim to open readers' minds to the critically divergent views that comprise our world's most important debates.

Introducing Issues with Opposing Viewpoints simplifies for students the enormous and often overwhelming mass of material now available via print and electronic media. Collected in every volume is an array of opinions that captures the essence of a particular controversy or topic. Introducing Issues with Opposing Viewpoints books embody the spirit of nineteenth-century journalist Charles A. Dana's axiom: "Fight for your opinions, but do not believe that they contain the whole truth, or the only truth." Absorbing such contrasting opinions teaches students to analyze the strength of an argument and compare it to its opposition. From this process readers can inform and strengthen their own opinions, or be exposed to new information that will change their minds. Introducing Issues with Opposing Viewpoints is a mosaic of different voices. The authors are statesmen, pundits, academics, journalists, corporations, and ordinary people who have felt compelled to share their experiences and ideas in a public forum. Their words have been collected from newspapers, journals, books, speeches, interviews, and the Internet, the fastest growing body of opinionated material in the world.

Introducing Issues with Opposing Viewpoints shares many of the well-known features of its critically acclaimed parent series, Opposing Viewpoints. The articles are presented in a pro/con format, allowing readers to absorb divergent perspectives side by side. Active reading questions preface each viewpoint, requiring the student to approach the material thoughtfully and carefully. Useful charts, graphs, and cartoons supplement each article. A thorough introduction provides readers with crucial background on an issue. An annotated bibliography points the reader toward articles, books, and Web sites that contain additional information on the topic. An appendix of organizations to contact contains a wide variety of charities, nonprofit organizations, political groups, and private enterprises that each hold a position on the issue at hand. Finally, a comprehensive index allows readers to locate content quickly and efficiently.

Introducing Issues with Opposing Viewpoints is also significantly different from Opposing Viewpoints. As the series title implies, its presentation will help introduce students to the concept of opposing viewpoints, and learn to use this material to aid in critical writing and debate. The series' four-color, accessible format makes the books attractive and inviting to readers of all levels. In addition, each viewpoint has been carefully edited to maximize a reader's understanding of the content. Short but thorough viewpoints capture the essence of an argument. A substantial, thought-provoking essay question placed at the end of each viewpoint asks the student to further investigate the issues raised in the viewpoint, compare and contrast two authors' arguments, or consider how one might go about forming an opinion on the topic at hand. Each viewpoint contains sidebars that include at-a-glance information and handy statistics. A Facts About section located in the back of the book further supplies students with relevant facts and figures.

Following in the tradition of the Opposing Viewpoints series, Greenhaven Press continues to provide readers with invaluable exposure to the controversial issues that shape our world. As John Stuart Mill once wrote: "The only way in which a human being can make some approach to knowing the whole of a subject is by hearing what can be said about it by persons of every variety of opinion and studying all modes in which it can be looked at by every character of mind. No wise man ever acquired his wisdom in any mode but this." It is to this principle that Introducing Issues with Opposing Viewpoints books are dedicated.

Introduction

"The persistent animal-welfare questions of our day center on institutional cruelties—on the vast and systematic mistreatment of animals that most of us never see."

— Matthew Scully, author of *Dominion: The Power of Men, the Suffering of Animals, and the Call to Mercy*

Upton Sinclair's famous 1906 book *The Jungle* featured a vivid portrayal of a meat-packing factory. His book, based on months of research, described rats being accidentally blended into sausage-grinding machines, spilled guts and dirt being swept off the floor and processed into meats, and other gruesome details. *The Jungle* became a bestseller and helped spur the federal government to pass the Food and Drug Act, setting federal government standards for meat for the first time. Interestingly, these results were not exactly what Sinclair was aiming for. He had hoped his book would expose people to the plight of poor immigrant workers in meat-packing plants, but the American public instead was fixated on the contents of their food. "I aimed at the public's heart, and by accident I hit it in the stomach,"[1] he once said.

A century later, similar questions are being raised by animal rights activists about the food on American dinner plates. But today's activists aim to focus public outrage not on the plight of workers, but on the plight of the animals themselves. Their campaigns are targeted at the vast majority of meat-eating Americans. Animal rights organizations have sought to raise public awareness of the way animals are treated in the food industry by providing graphic descriptions and photographs of how animals are bred, raised, and killed.

Efforts by People for the Ethical Treatment of Animals (PETA), for example, focus on how chickens are treated in the poultry industry. In recent years PETA activists have publicly demonstrated in front of restaurant chains such as McDonald's, Burger King, and Kentucky Fried Chicken (KFC). They have used brochures, undercover videos, and costumed demonstrators to publicize and condemn practices they

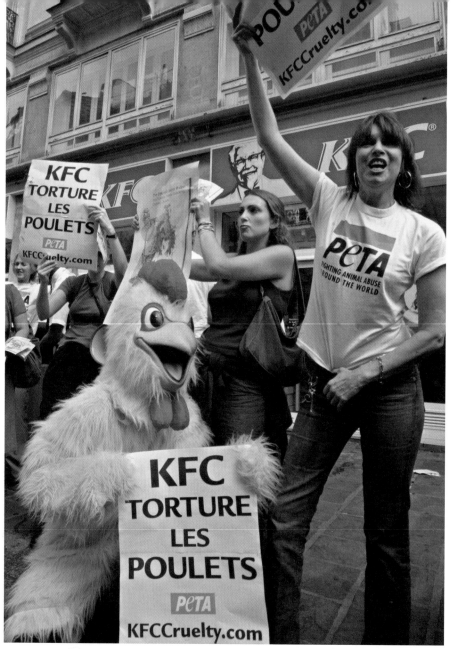

Animal rights activists protest in front of a KFC restaurant in Paris, France. Their signs read, "KFC tortures chickens."

view as inhumane. These include cutting off chicken's beaks, keeping hens in stacked cages as little as twenty inches wide (less than their natural wingspan), and killing chickens by slitting their throats and dumping them in boiling water to remove their feathers. PETA's campaigns have sought to change the behavior of both food consumers and restaurant chains. "If people know what happened to those chickens," says PETA spokesperson Bruce Friedrich, "raising them in their own filth, and then dumping them on an assembly line to have their throats cut when they're still alive, they wouldn't go to Kentucky Fried Chicken."[2] Friedrich's statement indicates that PETA's activities, like Upton Sinclair's book, is aimed not only at the heart, but also the stomach.

Another animal rights organization taking this tactic is the Humane Society of the United States (HSUS). HSUS has maintained that the crowded and unsanitary conditions many chickens live in can spread disease, cause stress for the chickens—and also pose a health risk to humans. According to Michael Greger of the HSUS, "by handling meat that is the product of an inhumanely slaughtered bird, consumers may well be at an increased risk for contracting a potentially life-threatening food-borne illness."[3]

The campaigns of PETA and HSUS have had some success in changing some food industry practices. McDonald's announced in 2000 that it would buy eggs from farms that treated hens more humanely. It also

Chickens on this organic farm in England are allowed to roam freely instead of being kept in cages.

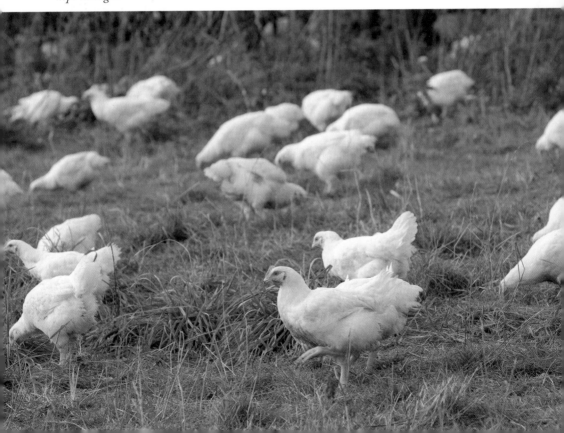

pledged to study the feasibility of using gas to kill chickens—something Greger and other animal advocates consider painless and safe. KFC has pledged to study and promote these kinds of humane practices among its meat suppliers, and similar concessions have been made by Burger King and other restaurant chains.

The concerns raised by PETA and other animal rights activists may also have had some effect on the eating habits of Americans. Some people have chosen to forgo meat and animal products altogether, or reduce such consumption in favor of meat and dairy substitutes such as soy milk. Others have chosen to pay higher prices for chicken and other meat and dairy products from operations that avoid controversial farming practices altogether. They buy chicken and eggs from smaller farms that do not use hormones and antibiotics on their animals, and raise cage-free chickens, for example. *Nutrition Business Journal* has estimated that such sales of "natural" meat, fish, and poultry reached $763

Members of People for the Ethical Treatment of Animals (PETA) protest against the mistreatment of circus animals.

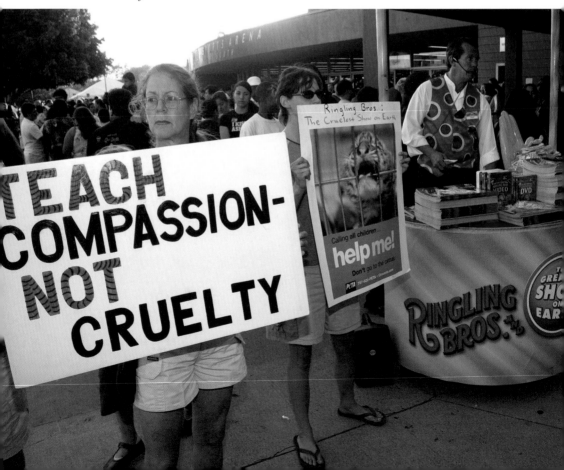

million in 2002—less than 1 percent of the total market, but a significant increase from previous years.

Food is just one of the many ways humans use animals. Animals are also used in the production of steel, rubber, and plastic goods, in medical experiments, and for companionship and entertainment. *Introducing Issues with Opposing Viewpoints: Animal Rights* presents debates in these different areas. In many cases both proponents and opponents of animal rights assume that treating animals better necessarily means humans must make inconvenient or impossible sacrifices. However, the success PETA and HSUS have had with their chicken campaigns indicates that in some cases people can be persuaded that it is in their own self-interest to care about the welfare and well-being of animals.

Notes
1. Upton Beall Sinclair Jr., *Dictionary of American Biography, Supplement 8: 1966–1970.* American Council of Learned Societies, 1988.
2. Quoted in Elizabeth Becker, "Group Says It Will Begin Boycott Against KFC," *New York Times*, January 6, 2003.
3. Humane Society of the United States press release, "The HSUS Files Lawsuit Challenging USDA's Exclusion of Birds from the Humane Methods of Slaughter Act," November 21, 2005.

Chapter 1

Do Animals Have Rights?

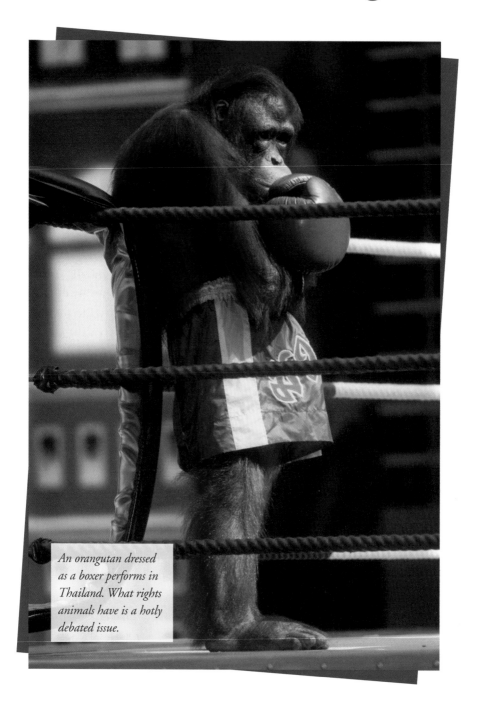

An orangutan dressed as a boxer performs in Thailand. What rights animals have is a hotly debated issue.

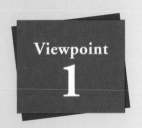
Animals Should Be Entitled to Rights

"It's past time for American justice to recognize that animals . . . have lives and interests of their own."

Animal Legal Defense Fund

The Animal Legal Defense Fund (ALDF) is a nonprofit organization of attorneys and activists who argue in the courts on behalf of particular animals. ALDF also works for political and legal reforms to promote animal rights. In the following viewpoint they explain why they believe that animals should be entitled to certain legal rights and protections. Billions of animals are cruelly mistreated and killed every year in part because they have the legal status of inanimate objects, according to the organization. ALDF argues that while nonhuman animals are not *people*, that does not mean animals cannot be treated as *persons* in the eyes of the law.

AS YOU READ, CONSIDER THE FOLLOWING QUESTIONS:
1. Do the authors believe that bacteria should have rights?
2. What entities, besides human beings, are considered legal "persons," according to ALDF?
3. According to ALDF, how many animals are killed each year for food in the United States?

If you've never given much thought to the concept of legal rights for animals—or if you've heard about it mainly from its more vocal opponents—the idea may strike you as frivolous, worrisome or just plain puzzling. Indeed, the very notion is a feast for fearmongers, who, while always careful to assert their support for animal *welfare*, just can't shake their nagging concerns about animal *rights*.

Bacteria Rights?

For instance:

- Isn't giving rights to animals a slippery slope?
- If these people get their way, would rights also be extended to, say, bacteria?
- Would chimps be allowed to vote in school board elections?
- When animals have rights, will I have to release Fido and Fluffy in the nearest national park, to commune with coyotes and mountain lions?

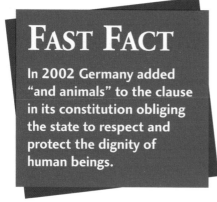

The Difference Between "People" and "Person"

To address these questions in order: No, no, no and no. Let's take a deep breath. Even the most hard-line advocates of animal rights—that is, those who insist on the total and immediate end of all forms of exploitation—recognize that nonhuman animals are not *people*. (Nor are they *things*, about which more in a moment.) But can animals be "persons"? That's a different matter.

Under U.S. law, Enron is a "person." So are WorldCom, Global Crossing, Adelphia Communications, accounting giant Arthur Andersen and virtually every other corporation in America, from tobacco firms to automakers to shopping mall developers. Your furry, flesh-and-blood friend, by contrast, is not only denied the personhood status enjoyed by these fictitious entities, but is treated by the

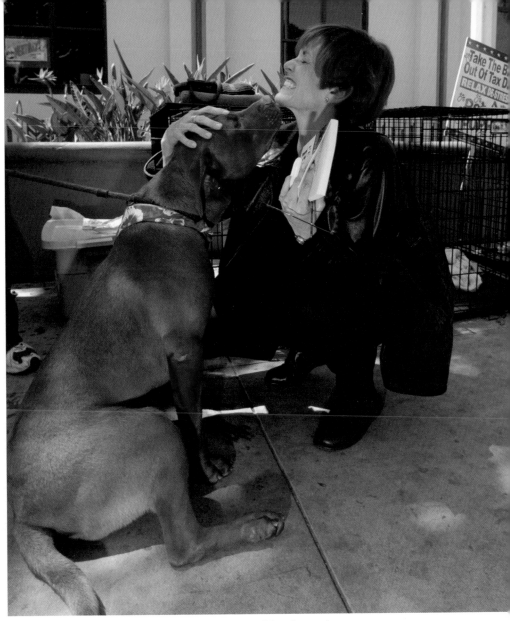

Many people treat their dogs and other pets as beloved family members.

courts as the equivalent of an inanimate object, like a chair or a piece of stereo equipment.

And that's simply wrong.

Justice for Animals

As advocates of legal rights for animals see it, animals' property status is what makes their exploitation possible—and changing that

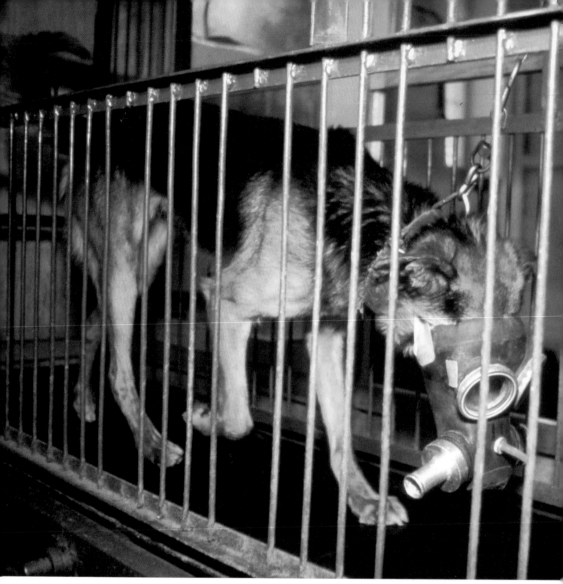

This dog was the subject of repeated chemical tests conducted at a Russian chemical weapons research facility.

status, therefore, is the key to ensuring that their interests are protected. Anti-cruelty laws notwithstanding, we still slaughter some 10 billion animals for food in the United States each and every year, under frequently appalling conditions. We hunt 200 million animals annually, and kill another 20 million in research and testing. And should someone maliciously kill your beloved companion animal, in most states all you could recover is the so-called "replacement value" of the animal—which, for that lovable mutt or tabby brought home from the shelter, is effectively zero. You could no more sue for emotional distress or loss of companionship than if someone destroyed your stereo.

It's past time for American justice to recognize that animals—in dramatic contrast to consumer products and faceless corporate entities—have lives and interests of their own. As with human rights under the law, these interests do not exist in a vacuum, but must be weighed against other, competing interests. (Or, in the words of a famous judicial axiom: Your right to swing your fist ends at the tip of my nose.) Our chief objective, as animal lawyers, is that the unmistakable interests of nonhuman animals be acknowledged under the law, and that humans be permitted to argue those interests in court.

This can only happen, however, when animals' status is elevated from property to something that more accurately reflects the current state of scientific knowledge and plain common sense.

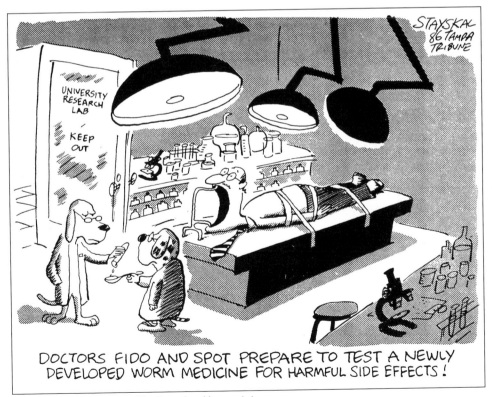

DOCTORS FIDO AND SPOT PREPARE TO TEST A NEWLY DEVELOPED WORM MEDICINE FOR HARMFUL SIDE EFFECTS!

Stayskal. © 1986 by Knight Ridder. Reproduced by permission.

Animals Are Not "Things"

It's impossible to predict precisely how America's courts might balance the interests of humans and nonhumans a century from now. For the moment, however—while chimps are still subject to legal captivity and torture in research labs, and the family dog's worth is set at the price of a video rental—we wouldn't worry too much about legal rights for bacteria. There's too much genuine misery here in the real world.

Let's start by simply recognizing that animals are not "things," and move on from there.

EVALUATING THE AUTHORS' ARGUMENTS:

The ALDF considers it wrong to view animals as "things." What do you think? Should animals be entitled to the rights and protections the authors describe? Explain your answer.

Animals Are Not Entitled to Rights

Edwin A. Locke

In the following viewpoint Edwin A. Locke argues that the concept of rights is meaningless to animals. In his opinion, human rights should apply only to creatures capable of grasping morality and engaging in rational thought. But animals, Locke maintains, cannot reason or learn a code of ethics, and thus are not entitled to the rights enjoyed by humans. Locke also accuses animal rights activists, including members of People for the Ethical Treatment of Animals (PETA), of harboring prejudice against humans.

Locke is a professor of business management at the University of Maryland at College Park and a senior writer for the Ayn Rand Institute, an organization that promotes the ideas of the late philosopher Ayn Rand.

> *"Rights are ethical principles applicable only to beings capable of reason and choice."*

AS YOU READ, CONSIDER THE FOLLOWING QUESTIONS:

1. According to the author, why is a lion not immoral for attacking a zebra?

2. According to Locke, what would PETA think of a cure for
   AIDS that had been discovered through animal research?
3. What does Locke believe to be the underlying motive of animal
   rights activists?

Human life versus animal life. This fundamental conflict of values, which was dramatized a few years ago when AIDS victims marched in support of research on animals, is still raging. PETA (People for the Ethical Treatment of Animals) has just launched a campaign against Covance, Inc., a biomedical research lab in Vienna, VA, that uses animals for drug testing.

It is an indisputable fact that many thousands of lives are saved by medical research on animals. But animal rightists don't care. PETA makes this frighteningly clear: "Even if animal tests produced a cure for AIDS, we'd be against it." Such is the "humanitarianism" of animal rights activists.

How do these advocates try to justify their position? As someone who has debated them for years on college campuses and in the media, I know firsthand: . . .

Men feel pain and have rights;
Animals feel pain;
Therefore, animals have rights.

This argument is entirely specious, because man's rights do not depend on his ability to feel pain; they depend on his ability to think.

Rights and Rationality

Rights are ethical principles applicable only to beings capable of reason and choice. There is only one fundamental right: a man's right to his own life. To live successfully, man must use his rational faculty—which is exercised by choice. The choice to think can be negated only by the use of physical force. To survive and prosper, men must be free from the initiation of force by other men—free to use their own minds to guide their choices and actions. Rights protect men against the use of force by other men.

Some critics argue against the idea of animal rights because animals, such as this lion feeding on a zebra, lack the ability to think rationally.

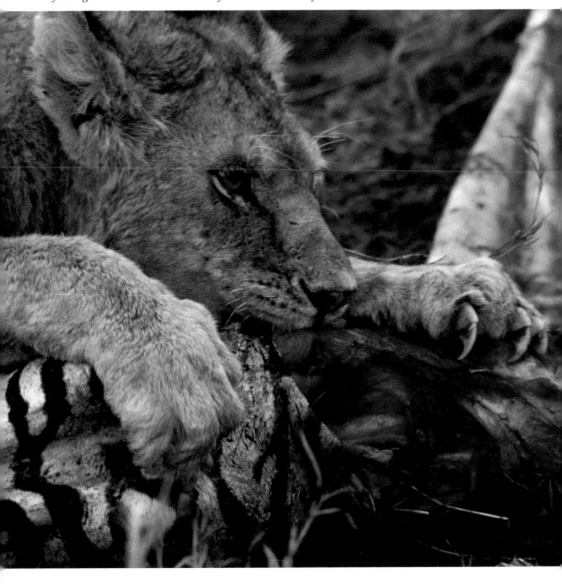

None of this is relevant to animals. Animals do not survive by rational thought (nor by sign languages allegedly taught to them by psychologists). They survive through sensory-perceptual association and the pleasure-pain mechanism. They cannot reason. They cannot learn a code of ethics. A lion is not immoral for eating a zebra (or even for attacking a man). Predation is their natural and only means of survival; they do not have the capacity to learn any other.

Only man has the power, guided by a code of morality, to deal with other members of his own species by voluntary means: rational persuasion. To claim that man's use of animals is immoral is to claim that we have no right to our own lives and that we must sacrifice our welfare for the sake of creatures who cannot think or grasp the concept of morality. It is to elevate amoral animals to a

An animal rights activist in France demonstrates against the use of animal fur for clothing.

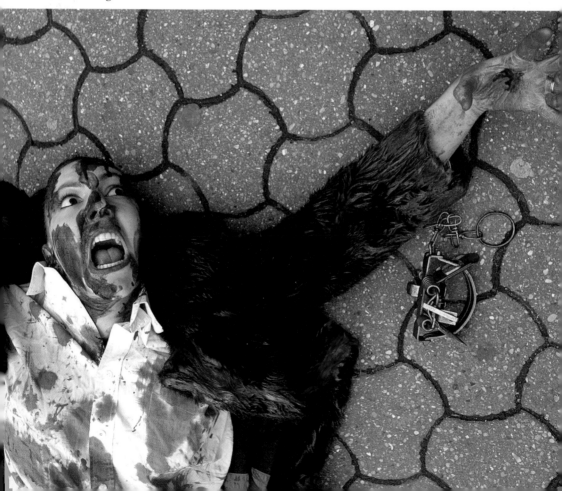

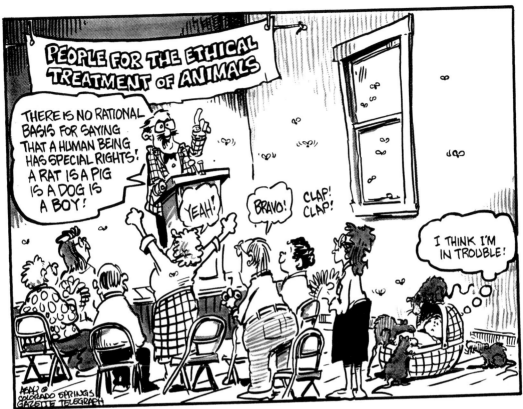

Asay. © by Chuck Asay. Reproduced by permission.

moral level higher than ourselves—a flagrant contradiction. Of course, it is proper not to cause animals gratuitous suffering. But this is not the same as inventing a bill of rights for them—at our expense.

The True Motives of Animal Rights Activists

The granting of fictional rights to animals is not an innocent error. We do not have to speculate about the motive, because the animal "rights" advocates have revealed it quite openly. Again from PETA:

- "Mankind is the biggest blight on the face of the earth";
- "I do not believe that a human being has a right to life";
- "I would rather have medical experiments done on our children than on animals."

These self-styled lovers of life do not love animals; rather, they hate men. . . .

They are not idealists seeking justice, but nihilists seeking destruction for the sake of destruction. They do not want to uplift mankind, to help him progress from the swamp to the stars. They want mankind's destruction; they want him not just to stay in the swamp but to disappear into its muck.

There is only one proper answer to such people: to declare proudly and defiantly, in the name of morality, a man's right to his life, his liberty, and the pursuit of his own happiness.

EVALUATING THE AUTHOR'S ARGUMENTS:

Edwin A. Locke argues that because animals cannot reason or follow a code of ethics, they do not deserve rights. Animal rights activists sometimes counter this logic by saying that some humans, such as the severely retarded or the comatose, do not have these abilities either, yet they have rights. What is your opinion of this debate? Does it affect whether you believe animals should or should not have rights?

Pets Should Have Some Rights

Lawrence Carter-Long

"The word 'owner' is outdated and doesn't reflect the human/ animal bond."

Should pets be more than just the property of their owners? In recent years several cities and states have passed legislation incorporating the term *animal guardian* into local laws governing pets and pet ownership. Lawrence Carter-Long writes in the following viewpoint that such a distinction can help elevate the status of animals and lead to better treatment for the nation's pets. It is important, Carter-Long says, for people to recognize that they have a responsibility to act as "guardians" of their animal companions. Carter-Long works for In Defense of Animals, an animal rights advocacy group that has campaigned for reforms in pet laws.

AS YOU READ, CONSIDER THE FOLLOWING QUESTIONS:

1. What are some of the cities that have incorporated the term *guardian* into their animal laws, according to the article?
2. What percent of households consider their pets to be "family members," according to the author?
3. According to Carter-Long, how does changing words affect a person's thought and actions?

As of this writing [January 2004] seven cities, Boulder, CO; San Francisco, West Hollywood and Berkeley, CA; Sherwood, AR; Menomonee Falls, WI; Amherst, MA; and the state of Rhode Island have officially recognized the important part animal companions play in our society by passing legislation that incorporates the term "guardian" into all their animal related ordinances.

The effort, launched by In Defense of Animals in 1999, was inspired by the belief that the term "animal guardian" instills a greater level of respect, responsibility and compassion towards the animals with whom we share our lives than the more commonly used phrase animal "owner."

Animals Are "Family Members"

Over 100 million dogs and cats are estimated to live in homes across our nation. A poll of 1,269 people last year [2003] revealed that a

This specialty store provides all-natural gourmet treats for pets. Pet supplies and services are a thriving industry in the United States.

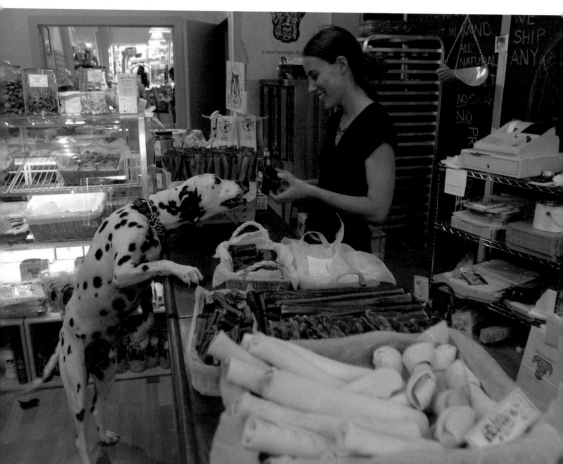

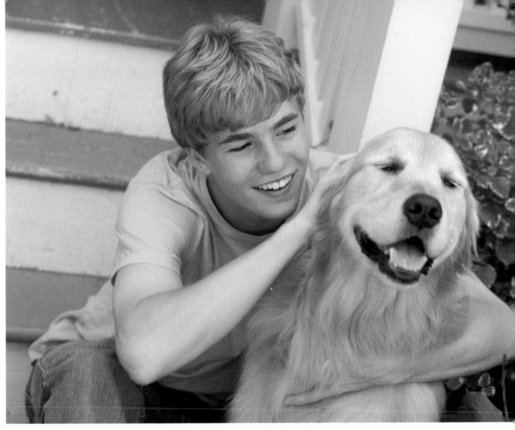

Dogs are kept as pets in millions of households across the United States.

whopping 97 percent planned to buy holiday gifts for their companion animals. Furthermore, 12 percent of those polled had returned previous gifts because their animal companions "did not like them." But, even in non-animal households, animals hold a special place in our hearts. Sixty-seven percent of surveyed respondents, including people with no animal companions, have helped a lost animal, or donated to an animal welfare organization.

At the University of Pennsylvania, social work services have been available since 1978 to those who have suffered the loss of an animal and an estimated one million dogs in the U.S. have been named the primary beneficiary in their guardian's will, so it should come as no surprise that animals are "family members" to at least 80 percent of the households who have them, according to one estimate.

More than Property

If these polls are any indication, dogs and cats are clearly much more than property, objects or things to most people, and as such, proponents of the "guardian" campaign highlight the necessity of updating our language to more accurately reflect this unique relationship.

"The word 'owner' is outdated and doesn't reflect the human/animal bond that exists in our culture today," says Jan McHugh, Executive Director of the Humane Society of Boulder Valley. "[Use of] the word 'guardian' denotes a higher level of responsibility towards another being. Although it is a simple language change, we hope . . . increased awareness of the 'guardian' language will elevate the status of animals in our community. We will use the word 'guardian' as another tool to fight animal abuse and exploitation."

The Power of Language

Words have power. How we think and talk is a precursor to how we act. By adjusting our language, we plant important seeds that influence future behavior. Updating city codes to include the term "animal guardian" means we're a step closer to recognizing the unique responsibility humans have in assuring an animal's care and well-being. While revising outmoded terminology does not alter one's legal rights, responsibilities and/or liabilities, the psychological and sociological impact of revising our language advances our respect and responsibilities to companion animals.

In terms of animal suffering, that shift seems essential.

Ed Boks, former Director of the Maricopa County Animal Care and Control in Phoenix, AZ, and the new Executive Director of NYC Animal Care and Control agrees. "Everything we do to enhance the human-animal bond minimizes the likelihood of an animal being relinquished. I support 'guardianship' language as a powerful shift in the way we speak and think about the companion animals that share our lives. By truly understanding what it means to be a guardian, more animals will be adopted and rescued. The guardianship initiative is

> **FAST FACT**
>
> On March 7, 1997, three youths broke into a cat shelter in Iowa and killed or injured 27 cats with baseball bats. They were charged only with misdemeanor offenses of "destroying property" since the value of stray cats was deemed limited.

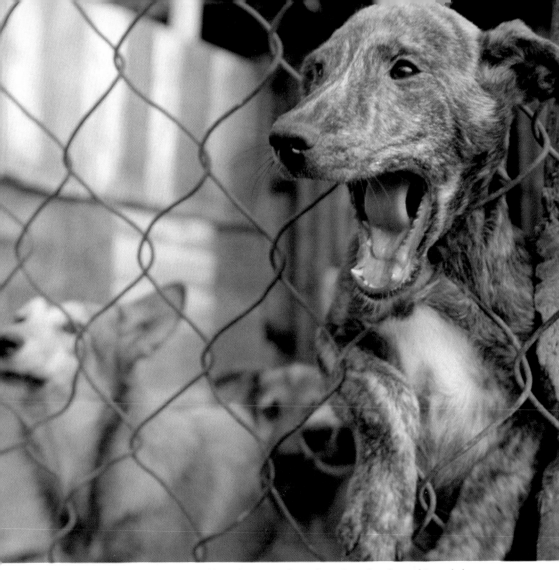

In the United States, millions of homeless animals, such as these dogs housed in a shelter, are euthanized each year.

leading to a better quality of life for animals as individuals, not as property."

To Reduce Abuse and Neglect

Carl Friedman, Director of the San Francisco Department of Animal Care and Control has stressed that, "It is my sincere belief that the result of increased numbers of people thinking and acting as 'guardians' of their animal companions will lead to fewer cases of abuse, neglect and abandonment and fewer animals being killed in our nation's shelters."

In a nation where between five to seven million homeless animals are killed annually, moving away from the notion that dogs and cats are mere property, objects and things—and as such, easily disposed of—is a core element of the campaign.

Boulder County's *Daily Camera* editorialized, "We're not declaring that all animals should be accorded the rights that humans should enjoy. But as people know intuitively, animals should be given more rights and respect than, say, a toaster." . . .

Compassion and Responsibility

The benefits of adopting guardian language and the behavior changes it can facilitate are far reaching, setting in motion greater transformations such as: Helping end the unnecessary deaths of millions of homeless animals in our nation's shelters, curtailing the abuse of animals by individuals and the puppy mill trade, better enforcement and strengthening of animal cruelty laws, and raising children to become compassionate and responsible adults.

What's in a word? Quite a lot.

EVALUATING THE AUTHOR'S ARGUMENTS:

Carter-Long includes quotations to support his argument. What kinds of sources does he quote? What effect do these quotations have on his argument, in your view? Explain.

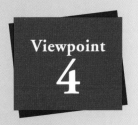

Pets Are Property

National Animal Interest Alliance

"Your right to own a pet could be at stake."

The National Animal Interest Alliance (NAIA) is an association of business, agricultural, scientific, and recreational interests dedicated to promoting animal welfare. In the following viewpoint the NAIA argues against the campaign to change local laws making pet owners "guardians." The organization argues that such a change would be a significant step toward granting animals legal rights. This would make veterinary care more expensive, lead to many lawsuits, and limit the rights of humans to own pets. NAIA charges that the real animal rights agenda is to eliminate pet ownership altogether, something that would be bad for both humans and animals.

AS YOU READ, CONSIDER THE FOLLOWING QUESTIONS:
1. What distinction does NAIA make between children and pets?
2. How much money do Americans spend on their pets each year, according to NAIA?
3. What specific laws does NAIA support?

"Animal guardian." It sounds innocent enough. Animal rights activists all across America are lobbying to change local laws so that pet owners become "guardians." The idea, they say, is to remind people that they are responsible for the animals in their care. But the agenda behind the guardian movement is to give animals legal standing to sue veterinarians, their owners, and others and to eventually end animal ownership altogether.

Parakeets and other bird species are kept as pets in at least 6 million U.S. households.

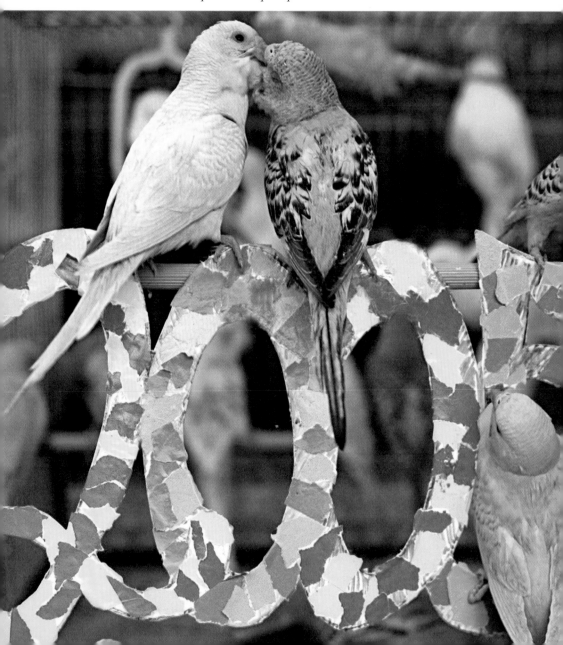

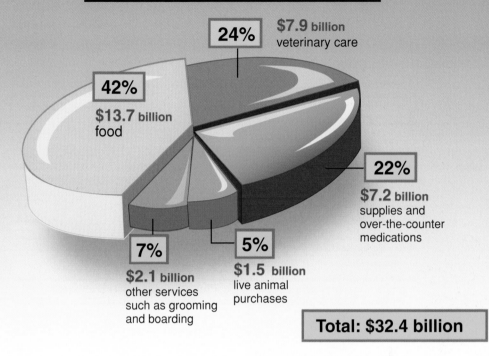

What Americans Spend on Pets

24% $7.9 billion veterinary care

42% $13.7 billion food

22% $7.2 billion supplies and over-the-counter medications

7% $2.1 billion other services such as grooming and boarding

5% $1.5 billion live animal purchases

Total: $32.4 billion

Source: American Pet Products Manufacturers Association, www.appma.org, April 22, 2004.

Activists Are Anti-Pet

Children need *guardians*. Pets need *owners*. Referring to dog owners as "guardians" means that people who buy dogs do NOT own them. Guardians care for the property of someone else. So, who will own pets if everyone is a guardian? The STATE?

Animal rights activists don't believe pets should be property. They reject the idea that human beings should have control over an animal's care, housing and training. The People for the Ethical Treatment of Animals Statement on Companion Animals says that animals should live their lives "free of human interference . . ." as "part of the ecological scheme." Ingrid Newkirk, PETA's co-founder, called pet ownership ". . . an absolutely abysmal situation brought on by human manipulation."

A First Step

NAIA strongly opposes the concept of legal guardianship for pets. Here's why: Changing the law so that pets are no longer property is really

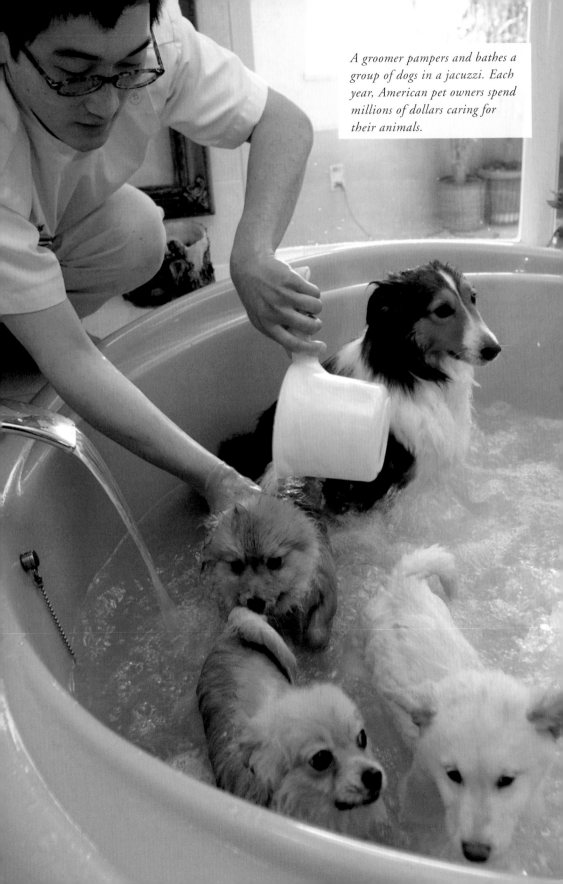

A groomer pampers and bathes a group of dogs in a jacuzzi. Each year, American pet owners spend millions of dollars caring for their animals.

the first step in the animal rights campaign to give animals the legal status of human beings.

Think for a moment about the practical consequences of giving human legal rights to animals:

- It will clog the courts with frivolous cases brought by animal rights extremists on behalf of dogs, cats and other pets.
- It will harm animals by creating confusion about who is responsible for their care.
- It will make veterinary care so expensive that many animals will not receive it or will be prematurely euthanized.
- It will lead to increasingly restrictive animal care laws and regulations.
- It will limit the right of individuals to buy and sell pets as they choose.

The animal rights campaign to end pet ownership is contrary to everything we know about American society. Americans believe in property ownership, and we own millions of pets. According to the American Pet Products Manufacturers Association, 62% of American households own at least one pet and 47% own more than one. These pet owners spend an estimated $30 billion annually on their dogs, cats, fish, birds, rodents and reptiles because they love their animals, and want to provide the best possible care for them.

FAST FACT

In July 2000, Boulder, Colorado, became the first U.S. city to replace all legal references to "pet owner" with "pet guardian."

The Bond of Ownership

Most pet owners consider their pets part of the family, but they also know that legal ownership makes them directly and legally responsible for pet care, protects pets from confiscation without cause, and preserves their rights to feed, house, train, care for and interact with their pets in ways that strengthen the human-animal bond.

Scientific research has confirmed the value of that bond to humans and animals alike.

NAIA strongly supports laws that preserve our right to own pets, recognize acceptable animal care practices based on sound veterinary science, clearly define animal cruelty and neglect, and hold animal owners fully accountable for animal welfare violations.

Normal Pets?

In the animal rights view, that's not enough. Wayne Pacelle, now vice-president of the Humane Society of the US, once said, "We have no problem with the extinction of domestic animals . . . one generation and out."

Another animal rights group said in a 1991 article, "Liberating our language by eliminating the word 'pet' is the first step. . . . In an ideal society where all exploitation and oppression has been eliminated, it will be (our) policy to oppose the keeping of animals as pets."[1]

The next time you hear animal rights activists calling for a guardianship change in local laws, pay close attention. Your right to own a pet could be at stake.

1. New Jersey Animal Rights Alliance, "Should Dogs Be Kept as Pets? NO!" *Good Dog!* Feb. 1991.

EVALUATING THE AUTHORS' ARGUMENTS:

In this viewpoint, the authors argue that laws changing the property status of pets will ultimately weaken the human-animal bond between pets and their owners. In the previous viewpoint, it was argued that such laws will strengthen and improve the bond between humans and their pets. Which viewpoint did you find more persuasive? Why?

Viewpoint 5

The Goals of Animal Rights Organizations Are Reasonable

Kathy Guillermo

"[PETA] will continue to do all it can legally and peacefully to give animals a voice."

Kathy Guillermo is a writer for People for the Ethical Treatment of Animals (PETA), a leading animal advocacy organization. In the following viewpoint she describes various campaigns PETA has undertaken to benefit animal welfare. PETA's undercover investigations have exposed animal cruelty in farms, laboratories, and circuses, she writes. It has also sponsored protests against grocery and fast food chains in order to compel these companies to improve the animal welfare practices of their suppliers. Guillermo pledges that PETA will continue fighting to help animals using legal and peaceful means.

AS YOU READ, CONSIDER THE FOLLOWING QUESTIONS:
1. What examples of cruelty to animals does Guillermo describe?
2. What are PETA's goals in its campaign against Kentucky Fried Chicken, according to the author?
3. What did PETA discover in its investigation of the University of North Carolina?

When People for the Ethical Treatment of Animals was founded more than 20 years ago, the term "animal rights" was relatively new. Most people thought little about the billions of animals raised and killed for food and clothing, experimented on in laboratories and caged in circuses. PETA's undercover investigations of deplorable conditions in laboratories and on factory farms shocked the public and lawmakers alike, and since then, animal-protection organizations have grown steadily larger and more successful in their efforts to rescue abused and neglected animals.

Animals have little protection under the law. The 10 billion animals raised for food every year in this country are routinely and legally mutilated—chicks have their beaks burned off while still alive, cows and pigs are castrated without anesthesia, cows are dehorned and branded—all without any painkillers. Most spend their lives confined to concrete stalls and metal cages in unnatural conditions. Some animals, such as veal calves, are kept in lonely isolation. Others, such as chickens, are crowded so closely together they can barely move.

Campaigns to Help Farm Animals

PETA campaigns to improve conditions for farmed animals. After PETA protested at more than 100 Safeway stores, the grocery chain became the first in U.S. history to improve conditions for the animals whose flesh it sells, pledging to increase space for laying chickens, to stop starving hens in order to force increased egg laying, and to conduct unannounced inspections of slaughterhouses and suppliers. PETA also persuaded Cincinnati-based Kroger, the nation's largest grocery chain, and Boise-based Albertson's, the second largest, to pledge to follow Safeway's lead. McDonald's, Burger King and Wendy's responded to PETA's campaign by making similar improvements.

PETA has now turned its attentions to Kentucky Fried Chicken. More than 700 million chickens raised each year for KFC are crammed by the tens of thousands into sheds that reek of ammonia fumes from accumulated waste. Each bird lives in the amount of space equivalent to a standard sheet of paper. They routinely suffer broken bones from being bred to be top-heavy, receive callous handling and are shackled

A PETA protester in the Philippines holds a sign that accuses KFC of animal cruelty.

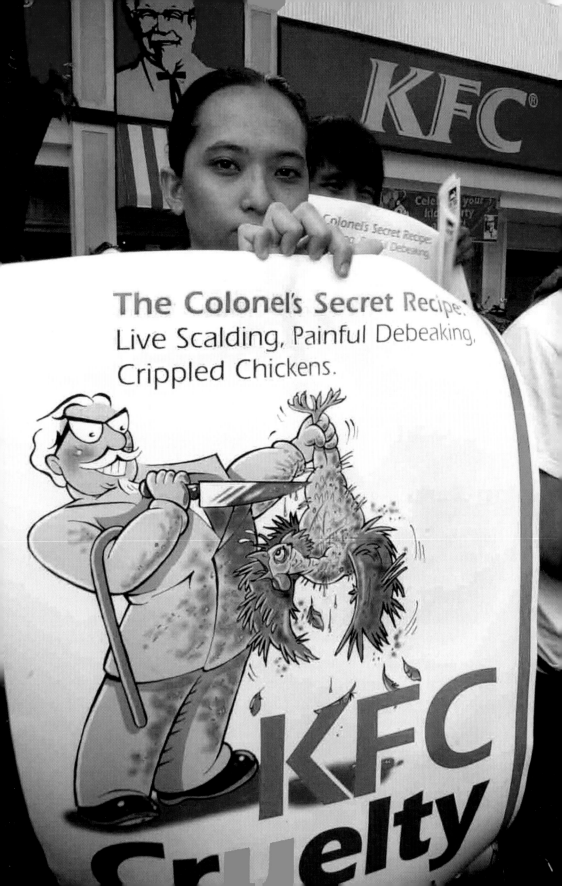

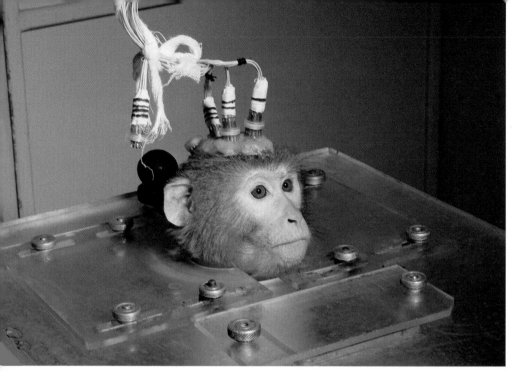

A monkey is restrained as a device measures its brain activity during a research experiment.

upside down at slaughterhouses. Chickens are often still fully conscious as their throats are slit or when they are dumped into tanks of scalding water to remove their feathers.

PETA is not seeking massive, industry-wide changes overnight. PETA simply asks that KFC commit to doing what it has promised: enact a comprehensive animal-welfare plan that will protect animals from abuse and neglect. These include replacing the present painful and traumatic slaughter methods with gas killing; mandating automated chicken catching using well-designed, gentle machines;[1] breeding birds for less aggression and healthier weights; and enriching the birds' barren living environments by simulating their natural habitats.

Exposing and Preventing Cruelty to Animals

Animals also suffer terribly in laboratories. Despite experimenters' claims that laboratory animals are protected by strict legislation, the Animal Welfare Act is the only federal law that covers the use of animals in experiments. It deals only with housing and maintenance stan-

---

1. According to PETA, using machines to catch chickens prevents injuries and stress that chickens experience when caught by hand.

dards. No laws exist preventing scientists from conducting painful or redundant experiments.

PETA has uncovered one case of cruelty after another. For example, an undercover investigation of the University of North Carolina's animal laboratories revealed multiple violations of regulations: cutting off live baby rats' heads with scissors without anesthesia, leaving live animals in cages with dead ones, failure to euthanize wounded and sick animals, and leaving hemophiliac mice with their tails cut off to bleed to death overnight. Following PETA's exposé, a supervisor resigned, scientists were disciplined and employee training strengthened. The

A circus elephant on parade in Chicago marches past a group of PETA demonstrators.

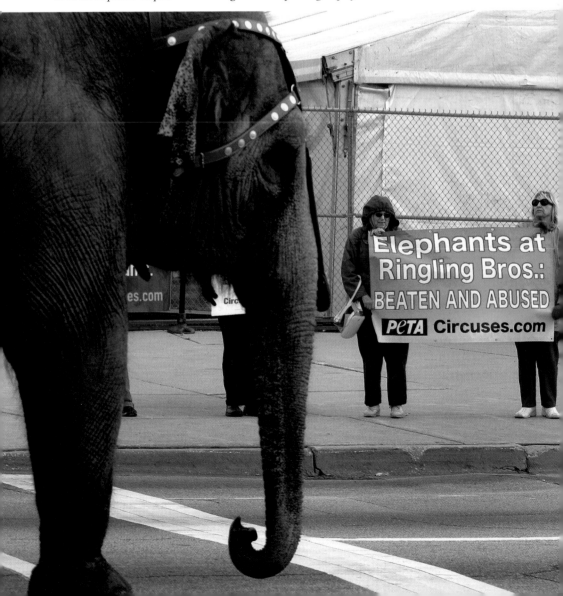

U.S. National Institutes of Health's office of Laboratory Animal Welfare has issued a new directive on euthanasia to all research institutions.

In circuses, animals are shackled and caged, dragged from town to town and forced to perform under threat of punishment. Enforcement of the few laws protecting these animals is often lax. It took many months for PETA to persuade U.S. and Puerto Rican officials to seize six thin, sick, lethargic, filthy polar bears from the traveling tropical Suarez Bros. Circus. PETA rallied support from polar-bear experts, Congress, and government officials in Germany and Canada. PETA's video footage showed the bears panting constantly while being hit, whipped and forced to perform frightening tricks in sweltering temperatures. A seventh bear had already been seized after PETA alerted the U.S. Fish and Wildlife Service about fraudulent documentation of its origin.

Giving Animals a Voice

While PETA is dedicated to exposing and ending abuses such as these, the organization has never supported or contributed—financially or otherwise—to violent or terrorist activities, though violence is committed against animals daily in the food, clothing, experimentation and entertainment industries. Despite the smear campaigns of some who feel threatened by the changes PETA's work brings, the organization will continue to do all it can legally and peacefully to give animals a voice.

EVALUATING THE AUTHOR'S ARGUMENTS:

Describe some of the specific practices regarding animal treatment the author wants to change. In your opinion, are these changes reasonable or radical? Explain your answer.

The Goals of Animal Rights Organizations Are Radical

AnimalScam.com

"The people who are doing the most to promote animal welfare . . . are the very ones that the animal rights movement wants to put out of business."

AnimalScam.com is a project of the Center for Consumer Freedom, a nonprofit organization supported by restaurants, companies, and individuals concerned about the animal rights movement. In the following viewpoint, AnimalScam.com argues that animal rights groups such as People for the Ethical Treatment of Animals (PETA) are radical organizations whose goals help neither animals nor people. The authors maintain that such groups seek to stop all human use of animals—a change they believe would drastically alter society and deprive people of such important items as food and medicine. "Liberating" all animals would also hurt animal welfare, AnimalScam.com contends, because it would end the livelihoods of farmers and others who are most involved in promoting the humane treatment of animals. The authors conclude that people who truly care about the welfare of animals should support local animal shelters and humane societies, and avoid patronizing animal rights organizations.

AS YOU READ, CONSIDER THE FOLLOWING QUESTIONS:
1. What phrase by PETA president Ingrid Newkirk sums up the goals of the animal rights movement, according to AnimalScam.com?
2. What violent tactics do the authors say are used by animal rights activists?
3. What are ten items animal rights activists want human consumers to do without, according to the authors?

Throughout most of history, human beings adopted more and more enlightened standards of animal "welfare" for their pets, livestock, and laboratory animals. Insisting on humane treatment for animals was an important economic decision. Farmers know that happy livestock animals produce more milk, better beef, and more valuable leather. Medical researchers know that their scientific work is meaningless without healthy lab animals. Animal welfare standards are just one way humans acknowledge the important bond between us and the animal world.

An Extremist Movement

But beginning in the second half of the twentieth century, activists lost their way. Instead of striving to strengthen this relationship by improving the lives of animals in our care, an extremist movement began attempting to terminate that connection entirely. Today, we call it the animal "rights" movement.

Animal-rights activists believe that animals should be completely separate from humankind. Their goal is to guarantee that the human race has absolutely no access to animals, no matter how important they may be for our survival and progress.

Ingrid Newkirk, co-founder and president of People for the Ethical Treatment of Animals (PETA), summed up the goal of today's modern animal rights movement in a recent speech. "Our goal," Newkirk told the Animal Rights 2002 convention, "is total animal liberation."

For the uninitiated, "total animal liberation" means permanently eliminating much of what we take for granted—regardless of how responsibly farmers, scientists, or trainers treat their animals. It may be hard to imagine a world without meat, eggs, leather, milk, or circuses; but there's no denying that animal-rights activists are gradually shifting these ordinary things to society's margins.

Violent Attacks

How? By consciously, shamelessly, viciously attacking people and businesses that don't subscribe to their "four legs good, two legs bad" world-view. Since the animal rights movement began gathering strength, over $100 million in property damage has been caused by animal-rights activists. A medical research executive was beaten with baseball bats. Countless death threats have been issued. Scientists have been sent razor blades in the mail. Trucks and buildings have been firebombed. Boats have been sunk.

Los Angeles police officers arrest animal rights demonstrators who allegedly vandalized the storefronts of fur stores during a 2000 protest.

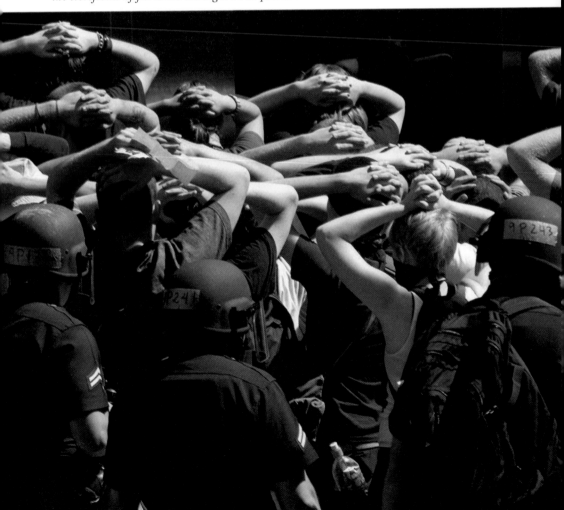

"People have died, and are going to die," said former Animal Liberation Front "spokesperson" . . . Kevin Kjonaas at the "Animal Rights 2002" convention. "This isn't a joke. It's not a game."

What Animals Provide for Humans

Here's just a partial list of what supporters of this violence-prone movement want us all to do without:

Food	Clothing	Sports & Entertainment
Bacon	Angora sweaters	Aquariums
Beef	Cashmere blazers	Bullfighting
Butter	Fur coats	Circuses
Cheese	Leather belts	Equestrian competition
Chicken	Leather jackets	Fishing
Eggs	Leather shoes	Greyhound racing
Hamburgers	Leather wallets	Horse racing
Honey	Silk scarves	Horse-drawn carriages
Kosher slaughter	Silk stockings	Hunting
Milk	Silk ties	Magic shows using animals
Milk chocolate	Wool scarves & mittens	Movies with animal actors
Omelets	Wool sweaters	Pet ownership
Pork	Worsted wool suits	Ranching
Turkey		Rodeos
Veal		Whaling
		Zoos

Science & Nature
Agricultural pesticides
Biology-class dissection
Fish farms
Medical research using animal test subjects
Surgical training using live animals

In the United States today, there are over 100 organizations dedicated to enforcing this animal "rights" mentality. Their annual budgets total more than $200 million. And they're deadly serious about achieving their goals.

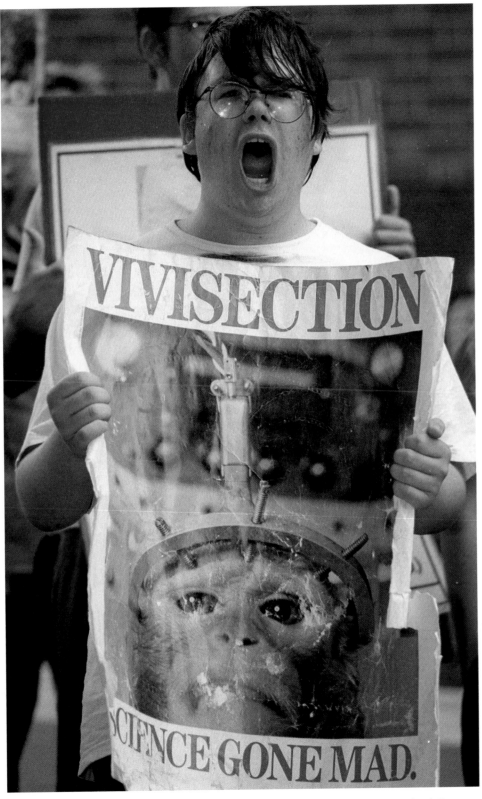

An activist protests animal research outside the University of Pennsylvania Medical Center at a 1999 demonstration.

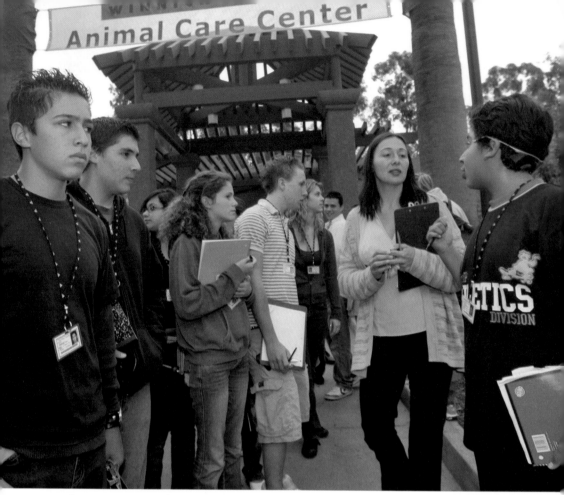

Some critics argue that animal-care centers such as this one in Los Angeles are more concerned with animal welfare than animal rights organizations.

People Who Care About Animal Welfare

In contrast, the people who are doing the most to promote animal welfare today are the very ones that the animal rights movement wants to put out of business.

Farmers can't survive without carefully-tended livestock. Many medical advances depend on the meticulous care given to lab animals. Anglers and hunters have a vested interest in the sustainability of animal populations that are vital to their sport. And millions of children learn important life lessons by visiting zoos and aquariums—and by loving and caring for dogs, cats, and other pets.

In a dishonest attempt to turn ordinary Americans against the responsible stewardship of animals, animal-rights activists have historically polluted the arena of ideas with shrill rhetoric, headline-grabbing stunts, and violent crimes. Their louder-is-better mentality threatens to further blur the line between animal welfare and animal rights. The consequences of this for our way of life would be disastrous.

If you want to support the humane treatment of animals, by all means support your local animal shelter, your local humane society (not the animal-rights-oriented Humane Society of the United States), or your local zoological park. It's true that animals deserve your help. But animal-rights organizations do not.

EVALUATING THE AUTHORS' ARGUMENTS:

The Center for Consumer Freedom receives much of its funding from restaurants, food companies, and others directly involved in practices opposed by animal rights activists. Does this background affect how you receive their arguments in this viewpoint? Why or why not?

Chapter 2

What Constitutes Ethical Treatment of Animals?

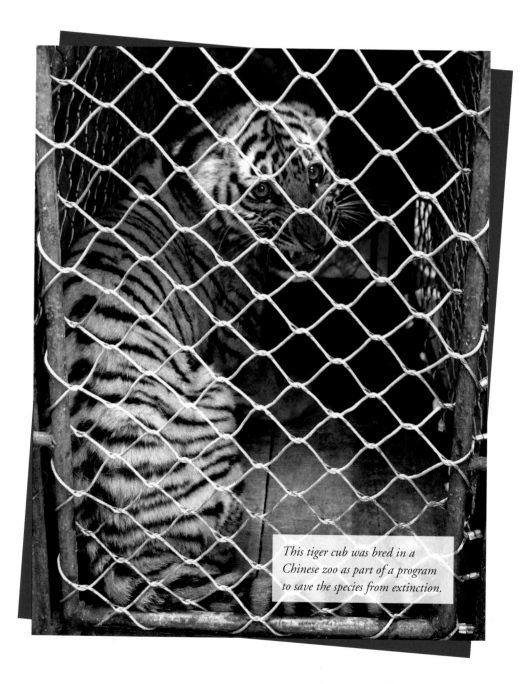

This tiger cub was bred in a Chinese zoo as part of a program to save the species from extinction.

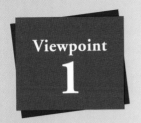

Eating Animals Is Wrong

Kim Scott

One of the primary ways humans use animals is for food. But some animal rights supporters contend that eating animals is similar to eating human flesh. The following viewpoint is taken from the winner of an essay contest held by the *Vegetarian Journal*. Kim Scott, age thirteen, writes that most of the meat people consume comes from factory farms and ranches in which animals are cruelly treated before they are slaughtered. She explains that she can no longer eat meat without thinking of the animal it once was. She expresses hope that future generations will come to view killing animals for food as immoral.

"Eating meat can no more be a 'choice' than can murder."

AS YOU READ, CONSIDER THE FOLLOWING QUESTIONS:

1. What circumstances led Scott to become a vegetarian?
2. What conditions do pigs and cows live in on factory farms, according to the author?
3. What are some of the challenges of being a vegetarian, according to Scott?

I t amazes me that most people are able to consume meat without thinking about the animal it recently was. We can look at a hamburger and see only a juicy, delicious American classic, not a fellow creature's suffering.

Making the Connection

I am a vegetarian because I can't put animals on one side of my brain and their cooked bodies on the other without connecting the two. When I see my father carving Thanksgiving dinner, I see the meat for what it is: the beheaded and disemboweled corpse of a specific turkey who was alive only days ago. I used to eat meat, but I had to make a conscious effort not to think about its source. I became less and less successful at this deception, and eventually I refused to eat meat altogether. Deciding to go vegetarian was as simple as making the connections that others refuse to think about until they find a blood vessel in a chicken nugget or have to dissect a cow's eye.

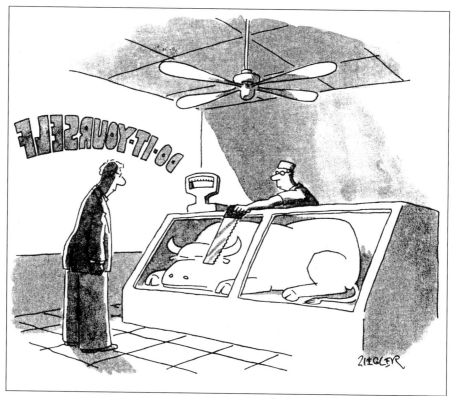

Ziegler. © 1984 by Cartoonbank.com. All rights reserved. Reproduced by permission.

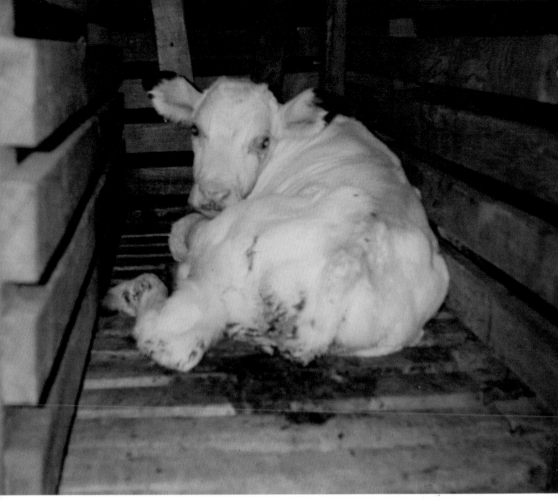

Calves raised for veal are kept immobilized in tiny crates. They frequently suffer from anemia, diarrhea, and other diseases.

Going vegetarian is as simple as realizing that meat comes from real animals. Even the neatly packaged meat at the supermarket is the muscle tissue of animals who were cruelly raised and slaughtered. The storybook image of a farm—a few cows grazing, perhaps with a cheery red barn in the distance—isn't accurate anymore. These days, many farm animals spend their lives in cramped cages on what have become known as factory farms. Efficiency is what counts there—not humane treatment. Animals are given as little space as possible. For cows and pigs, this often isn't enough to turn around! After their brief lives at the "factories," the animals are crammed into trucks. Many are injured or die slowly on the way to the "processing plants" where they are killed. Although pigs and cattle are supposed to be stunned before their throats are slit, reports say that some animals are fully conscious

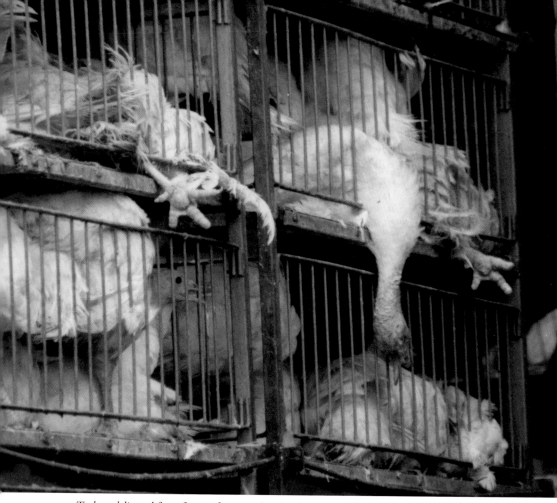

Turkeys delivered from factory farms to slaughterhouses are often transported in confining crates.

as they hang upside-down on conveyor belts, draining. Is a cheeseburger really worth this suffering?

Eating Meat Is Murder

Unfortunately, the problem is so far removed from our everyday life that most people just don't care. We don't have to look into the animals' eyes as they die; we don't even have to know who they were or what they went through. For more people to switch to a vegetarian diet, we will all have to think about—and care about—gruesome events taking place hundreds of miles away. Since that's not very much fun, it will be hard to effect this change in thinking. But we must make the effort, even if it seems futile sometimes, because we cannot allow the atrocities hidden in the farming industry to continue. Eating meat can no more be a "choice" than can murder. I hope that in eighty years, my grandchildren will be shocked to learn that you could get meat in a regular grocery store when I was little.

Sometimes it can be difficult to be a vegetarian, but for me, finding food to eat isn't the problem. Instead, the challenges lie in social situations. I am often the first vegetarian someone has met, so I feel a lot of pressure to give a good impression of vegetarians. I have to make sure that I don't insult my friends when I disagree with them and that I am polite when answering rather unreasonable arguments such as, "Vegetables can feel pain, too." and "But the animals are dead when we eat them!" At the same time, I want to make my beliefs known and educate others about how animals are treated. Balancing tact and activism can be hard, because although I don't think anyone should eat meat, I realize that an angry approach won't help.

All in all, though, I think that the advantages of being a vegetarian far outweigh the sometimes onerous responsibilities. By giving up meat I have ended my direct contribution to one of the worst forms of cruelty in all of history. I know that what I am doing is making a difference, and that eventually compassion and justice will prevail.

EVALUATING THE AUTHOR'S ARGUMENTS:

Consider the reasons the author gives for not eating meat. In your opinion, how persuasive is her argument? If you are a meat eater, has she convinced you to consider changing your diet? Why or why not?

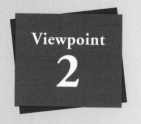

Eating Animals Is Not Wrong

Maxwell Goss

"The pleasure humans take in eating meat outweighs the suffering of the animals involved."

In the following viewpoint Maxwell Goss argues that it is ethical for humans to eat animals. He bases his argument on the idea that eating meat is a highly pleasurable activity. Furthermore, he says, cattle and other food animals do not suffer as much as some people believe. Therefore, he reasons, eating meat is not morally wrong. Goss is the founder and editor of Right Reason, a Web site devoted to conservative philosophical discussions.

AS YOU READ, CONSIDER THE FOLLOWING QUESTIONS:

1. What does the word *utilitarian* mean in the context of this viewpoint?
2. What constitutes a typical life of cattle, according to the author?
3. Does Goss believe humans can treat animals any way they want?

V egetarianism is sometimes justified on utilitarian grounds. One common line of argument goes something like this:

Humans and animals have a morally significant similarity, namely, the capacity for pleasure and pain, and they have no morally significant difference. Given this, there is no justification for automatically allowing the interests of humans to trump those of animals. Rather, humans must balance their interests against those of animals in deciding how they

An estimated 20 billion hot dogs were consumed in the United States in 2001—fifty of them by Takeru Kobayashi at a hot dog eating contest that year.

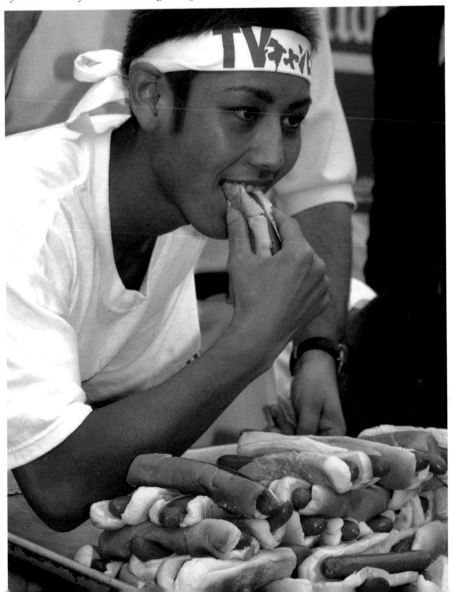

ought to treat them. But eating meat provides only a trivial pleasure to humans compared to the pain suffered by the animals eaten. Therefore, humans should not eat animals.

The Pleasure of Eating Meat

Discussion often centers on whether humans and animals have any morally significant difference, i.e. on whether, for instance, humans have rights and animals do not. I wish to set this important question aside and concentrate on the claim, which many vegetarians take for granted, that the pleasure of eating meat is trivial. Is it really? I, for one, derive quite a good

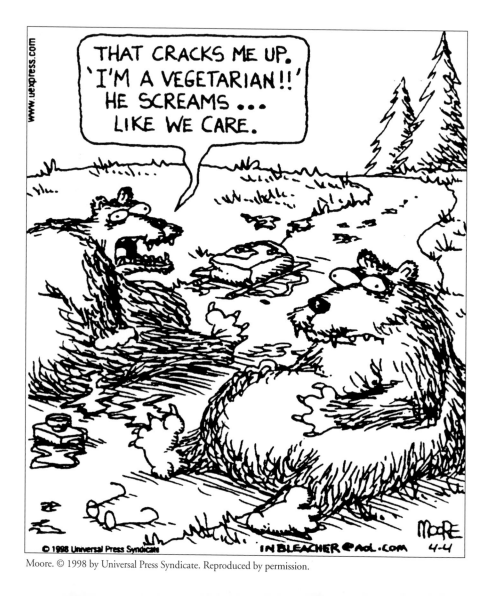

Moore. © 1998 by Universal Press Syndicate. Reproduced by permission.

deal of pleasure from consuming a rare New York strip steak, a half-pound of barbecued brisket, or a greasy cheeseburger at a corner bar. Moreover, meat is the most essential element in a ritual that brings a whole afternoon of pleasure to me and my guests alike: the backyard cook-out. I do not know how to quantify pleasures, but I do know how to rank them, and the pleasures just mentioned are not far from the top for me. And I am certainly not alone.

Now consider the life of a typical free-range Hereford heifer, a common sight throughout Texas and many other parts of the United States. This animal spends its life eating grass, moving from pasture to pasture, mooing, and standing around. I do not know much about the interior life of cattle, but these activities would seem to be the very definition of pleasure for such a beast. After maybe sixteen or eighteen months our heifer and its companions are herded into a feedlot, where they are fattened up for ninety days with corn or other high-calorie feed. Finally, our heifer is brought into the killing stall, where it is stunned and then, unconscious, bled to death. When done properly, the heifer feels only a moment's pain.

A normal head of cattle might yield in the neighborhood of eighty pounds of steak, eighty pounds of roast, and over one hundred pounds of ground beef, not to mention the tenderloin, ribs, and low-grade beef of various kinds. That is quite a few backyard cook-outs.

Given all this, it is hard to see how one could conclude that, in the example given, human pleasure is outweighed by animal displeasure. Moreover, inasmuch as the treatment of our heifer is not atypical in the cattle industry, it is clear that there are many real-world cases in which the butchering and eating of meat are quite justified on utilitarian grounds.

Objections and Replies

Some will object: What about factory farming? What about the cattle that are improperly stunned and are awake as the blood drains

> ## FAST FACT
>
> In 2002 total meat consumption (red meat, poultry, and fish) amounted to 200 pounds (90kg) per person in the United States, according to the U.S. Department of Agriculture.

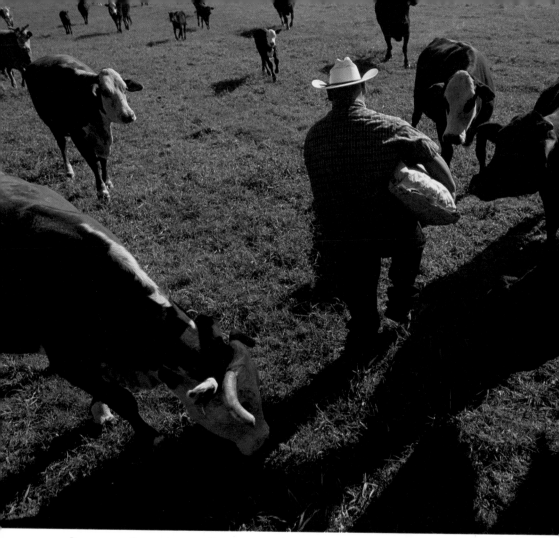

Proponents of a carnivorous diet maintain that cattle raised on ranches are well cared for and are not subjected to cruelty.

from them? My reply is that some current agricultural practices are indeed morally problematic. But this hardly invalidates my main point, which is that the utilitarian gives us no good reason to think that eating meat is not permissible in a significant range of cases.

Others will object: Similar pleasures are afforded by a vegetarian diet, which involves little or no animal suffering, and so there can be no justification for eating meat. My reply is that, having once been a serious vegetarian, I know that one can eat well on a meatless diet. However, I also know that a whole range of gustatory pleasures are unavailable to the vegetarian and that many people, myself included, find these far preferable to the meatless alternatives.

Cattle Pleasure and Pain

Still others will object: An eighteen-month old heifer does not merely experience momentary pain; it is also deprived of its future, with all its attendant pleasures and satisfactions. My reply is that the heifer would also have not had its past, with all its attendant pleasures and satisfactions, were it not for the demand for its meat. Ranching brings into the world at least as much cattle-pleasure as it takes out.

Finally, some will say: You would never make a similar argument for raising, slaughtering, and eating humans. My reply? Indeed I would not, because I hold that there is a morally significant difference between humans and animals. But this brings us back to the premise of the argument against eating meat that I have set aside. My present point is that, whatever the status of this premise, the pleasure/pain calculus does not give sufficient grounds for vegetarianism.

I hasten to add that nothing I have said here entails, or should be taken even to suggest, that one is permitted to treat animals in any way he wishes. Far from it; animals should be treated humanely. However, my argument does entail that what many vegetarians take to be obvious is actually empirically false. In many cases, the pleasure humans take in eating meat outweighs the suffering of the animals involved. Eating meat can be justified on utilitarian grounds.

EVALUATING THE AUTHOR'S ARGUMENTS:

How does Goss's description of what cattle experience differ from that of Scott in the previous viewpoint? Do you believe that a utilitarian measuring of pleasure and pain is an appropriate way to determine the morality of eating animals? Why or why not?

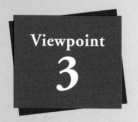

Zoos Violate Animals' Rights

People for the Ethical Treatment of Animals

"The idea of keeping animals confined behind cage bars is obsolete."

Liberty has long been understood as a fundamental human right. But some animal rights supporters believe that freedom should be granted to animals as well. The following viewpoint holds that zoos unjustly keep animals in captivity, away from their natural homes. It is taken from a fact sheet produced by People for the Ethical Treatment of Animals (PETA), an organization that fights for animal rights. PETA argues that being kept captive causes stress and mental problems for many animals. PETA also provides examples of how animals are beaten or otherwise mistreated in zoos.

AS YOU READ, CONSIDER THE FOLLOWING QUESTIONS:

1. What do zoos teach people about animals, according to the authors?
2. What is the condition PETA describes as "zoochosis"?
3. What response does PETA make to the claim that zoos help preserve endangered species?

Despite their professed concern for animals, zoos can more accurately be described as "collections" of interesting "specimens" than actual havens or simulated habitats (real homes). Zoos teach people that it is acceptable to interfere with animals and keep them locked up in captivity where they are bored, cramped, lonely, deprived of all control over their lives, and far from their natural homes. . . .

Zoos Hurt Animals

Zoos vary in size and quality—from drive-through parks to small roadside menageries with concrete slabs and iron bars. Although more

An orangutan confiscated from an animal market in Indonesia looks out from his cage at an animal shelter.

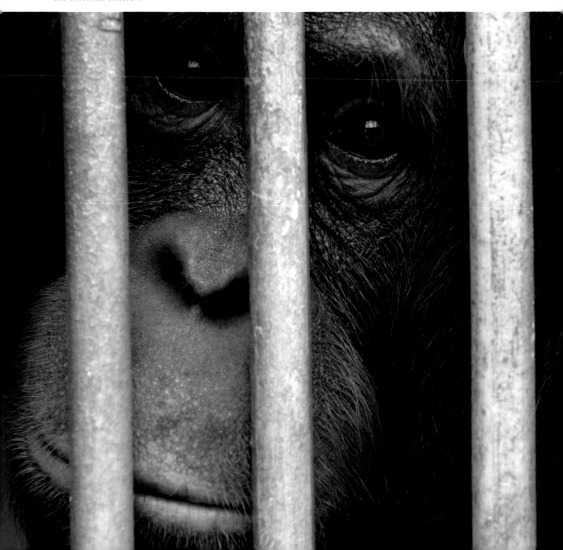

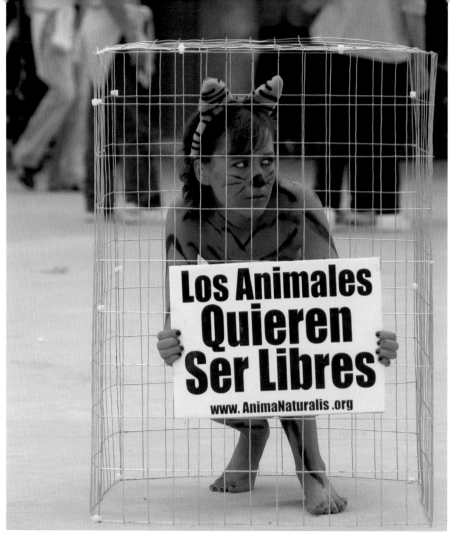

A PETA activist demonstrates against keeping wild animals in zoos. The sign reads, "Animals Want to Be Free."

than 135 million people visit zoos in the United States and Canada every year, most zoos operate at a loss and must find ways to cut costs or add gimmicks that will attract visitors. . . .

Ultimately, animals are the ones who pay the price. Precious funds that should be used to provide more humane conditions for animals are often squandered on cosmetic improvements, such as landscaping or visitor centers, in order to draw visitors.

Animals suffer from more than neglect in some zoos. Rose-Tu, an elephant at the Oregon Zoo, suffered "176 gashes and cuts" inflicted by a zoo handler wielding a sharp metal rod. Another elephant, Sissy, was beaten with an ax handle at the El Paso Zoo.

The animals on exhibit are not the only ones who suffer. Most zoos have an area that the public never gets to see, where rabbits, rats, mice, baby chicks, and other animals are raised and killed to provide food for the animals on display. According to one zoo volunteer, killing methods include neck-breaking and "bonking," in which zookeepers place "feed" animals in plastic bags and slam their heads against a hard surface to induce fatal head injuries.

Propagation, Not Education

Zoos claim to educate people and preserve species, but they usually fall short on both counts. Most zoo enclosures are very small, and rather than promoting respect or understanding of animals, signs often provide little more information than an animal's species, diet, and natural range. Animals' normal behavior is seldom discussed, much less observed, because their natural needs are rarely met. Birds' wings may be clipped so that they cannot fly, aquatic animals are often without adequate water, and many animals who live in large herds or family groups in nature are kept alone or, at most, in pairs. Natural hunting and mating behaviors are virtually eliminated by regulated feeding and breeding regimens. Animals are closely confined, lack privacy, and have little opportunity for mental stimulation or physical exercise. These conditions often result in abnormal and self-destructive behaviors or "zoochosis."

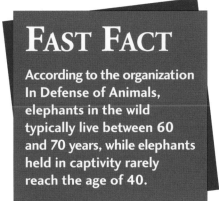

FAST FACT

According to the organization In Defense of Animals, elephants in the wild typically live between 60 and 70 years, while elephants held in captivity rarely reach the age of 40.

An Oxford University study based on four decades of observing animals in captivity and in the wild found that animals such as polar bears, lions, tigers, and cheetahs "show the most evidence of stress and/or psychological dysfunction in captivity" and concluded that "the keeping of naturally wide-ranging carnivores should be either fundamentally improved or phased out."[1] A PETA investigation of numerous

1. Ros Clubb and Georgia Mason, "Captivity Effects on Wide-Ranging Carnivores," *Nature*, October 2, 2003.

zoos across the country found that several bear species, including sun, grizzly, Kodiak, spectacled, black, and sloth bears, were exhibiting neurotic, stereotypic behaviors. These frustrated animals spend much of their time pacing, walking in tight circles, swaying or rolling their heads, and showing other signs of psychological distress. In some bear enclosures, paths worn by the bears' constant pacing can be seen; in others, there are actual paw impressions in the soil where bears have repeatedly stepped in the same spot. These behaviors are not just symptoms of boredom, they indicate profound despondency.

A polar bear at a zoo in New York looks out of her enclosure. Polar bears in captivity frequently exhibit symptoms of distress.

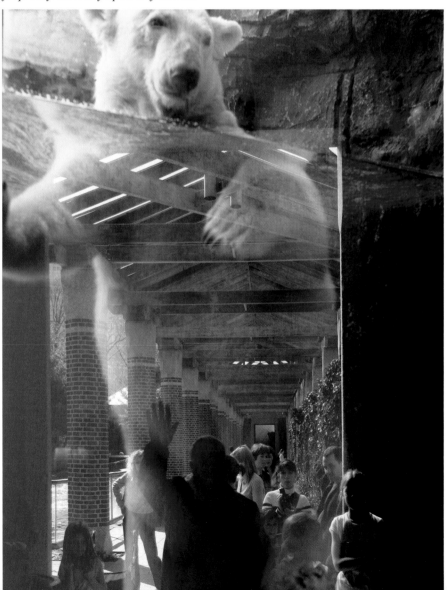

As for the claim that zoos provide educational opportunities—consider that most visitors spend only a few minutes at each display, seeking entertainment rather than enlightenment. . . .

The purpose of most zoos' research is to find ways to breed and maintain more animals in captivity. If zoos ceased to exist, so would the "need" for most of their research. Protecting species from extinction sounds like a noble goal, but zoo officials usually favor exotic or popular animals who draw crowds and publicity rather than threatened or endangered local wildlife. The Chinese government, for example, "rents" pandas to zoos worldwide for fees of more than $1 million per year, but some question whether the profits are being directed toward panda-conservation efforts at all.

Most animals housed in zoos are neither endangered nor being prepared for release into natural habitats. . . .

When Cute Little Babies Grow Up

Zoo babies are crowd-pleasers, but when they get older and attract fewer visitors, many are sold or killed by zoos. Deer, tigers, lions, and other animals who breed frequently are sometimes sold to "game" farms where hunters pay for the "privilege" of killing them; others are killed for their meat and/or hides. Other "surplus" animals may be sold to circuses or smaller, more poorly run zoos.

A chimpanzee named Edith is one example of a discarded zoo baby who fell into the wrong hands. Born in the 1960s at the Saint Louis Zoo, baby Edith was surely an adorable sight for visitors. But just after her third birthday, she was taken from her family and passed around to at least five different facilities, finally landing at a Texas roadside zoo called the Amarillo Wildlife Refuge (AWR). During an undercover investigation of AWR, PETA found Edith in a filthy, barren concrete pit. She was hairless and had been living on rotten produce and dog food. . . .

Another example involves Twiggs and Jeffrey, two giraffes born at the Cape May County Zoo. When they got older, they were sold by the zoo to a broker who subsequently sold them to a traveling circus. The director of the Cape May County Zoo actually admitted to seeing the animals' pitiful living conditions in the circus but did not have a problem with the situation. . . .

Beyond Zoos

Ultimately, we will only save endangered species by preserving their habitats and combating the reasons why they are killed by people. Instead of supporting zoos, we should support groups like the International Primate Protection League, the Born Free Foundation, the African Wildlife Foundation, and other groups that work to preserve habitats. We should help nonprofit sanctuaries that are accredited by The Association of Sanctuaries, such as the Elephant Sanctuary and the Performing Animal Welfare Society. These sanctuaries rescue and care for exotic animals without selling or breeding them.

With all the informative television programming, our access to the Internet, and the relative ease of international travel, learning about or viewing animals in their natural habitats can be as simple as a flick of a switch or a hike up a mountain. The idea of keeping animals confined behind cage bars is obsolete.

EVALUATING THE AUTHORS' ARGUMENTS:

PETA is an animal rights organization that opposes the use of animals for food, clothing, research, entertainment, or even pets. The author of the next viewpoint professionally evaluates and rates zoos. Does knowing the background of these authors influence your reading of their views? If so, in what way?

Well-Run Zoos Do Not Violate Animals' Rights

John Ironmonger

"Most zoo keepers . . . believe that animals in their charge are contented and as 'happy' as their wild relations."

John Ironmonger is the author of *The Good Zoo Guide*, a ratings guide to zoos in Great Britain. He helped found Goodzoos.com, a Web site featuring evaluations of zoos worldwide on how they treat their animals. In the following viewpoint he addresses the question of whether it is cruel to keep animals captive in zoos. He argues that in well-maintained zoos, animals typically live longer and are less prone to disease than animals in the wild. Captive animals also do not suffer from predators or famine. Furthermore, the concept of "freedom" is a human construct, he argues, that is not relevant to animals. Ironmonger concludes the zoos are continually improving how they treat their animals.

AS YOU READ, CONSIDER THE FOLLOWING QUESTIONS:

1. What is the position of the Royal Society for the Prevention of Cruelty to Animals regarding zoos?

I n the United Kingdom, The [Royal Society for the Prevention of Cruelty to Animals] RSPCA, guardian of Britain's conscience in these matters, is ambivalent in its attitude towards zoos. Officially it is neither pro-zoo, nor anti-zoo. Instead it claims to support good zoos and to oppose bad ones. Most zoo visitors are similarly even-minded about the issue. And yet the question is valid nonetheless. Is it possible that we have somehow become inured to the concept of animal captivity, in the same way perhaps as two centuries ago we might have accepted the concept of slavery, or as the Romans accepted the principle of human sacrifice as entertainment? Will future generations look back upon our own as barbaric because of our treatment of zoo animals?

Good Zoos and Bad Zoos

Like so many of the issues that surround zoos, a lot depends upon your assessment of the extremes. Who, for example, would take offence at the sight of a well-fed native pony grazing in an acre field? Few people would see cruelty there. Yet who would not feel sorry for a tiger in a circus trailer, endlessly pacing before the bars. By understanding that there is a spectrum of possible conditions of captivity from national parks to battery pigs, and by appreciating that we all have a threshold beyond which we will point the finger and say 'that is cruel', we can begin to delimit the types of zoos that we can accept. Of course there will be those who will condemn even the captive moorland pony, and for them no zoo will ever meet with their satisfaction. There is nothing wrong with this attitude. It is a perfectly rational point of view, and those that hold it are genuine animal lovers with a real concern for animal welfare.

But most zoo keepers are genuine animal lovers too. They believe that animals in their charge are contented and as 'happy' as their wild relations. Certainly zoo animals do tend to live longer lives, to feed better, and to suffer from fewer parasites or diseases. They live without the fear of predation; they live without famine. And the freedom, that they also live without, is seen by people like the late [naturalist] Gerald Durrell as a purely human construct, largely irrelevant to the day to day lives of animals.

Animals and Their Environment

So how should we determine whether a zoo enclosure is cruel or not? Zoologists can try to assess how similar the behaviour of a captive animal is to a wild animal of the same species—but it does not necessarily follow that, for example, a wolf that sleeps all day in a zoo cage is less happy than a hungry wild wolf whose time is spent searching for food. Similarly it may be unreasonable to assume that animals are happiest in an environment that mimics their own wild habitat. John Knowles of Marwell Zoo used to theorise that animals like the scimitar-horned oryx, which normally pick out a meagre existence in the semi-desert

Many zoos sponsor programs to breed animal species threatened with extinction. Here, handlers at a Chicago zoo observe a rare black rhinoceros calf born in 2003.

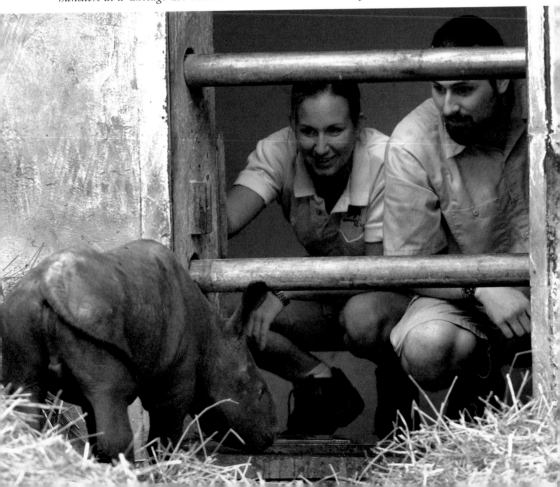

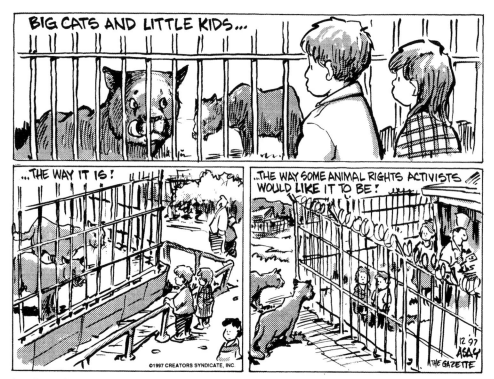

Asay. © 1997 by Creators Syndicate, Inc. Reproduced by permission.

scrubland of the Sahara, do so not because they choose or enjoy this harsh environment, but because they have been forced to the fringes by species better equipped to out-compete them elsewhere. According to this theory the scimitar-horned oryx should be in heaven among the lush meadows of southern England—as indeed they seem to be. The lions at zoos like Chester in the North of England are offered the option every winter day of centrally heated accommodation, or the chill winds of Cheshire. They virtually always choose to brave the elements, even preferring ice and snow to the warmth indoors—a reminder perhaps that although we think of lions as tropical animals, they once roamed throughout Europe, and their current range is directly due to human intervention.

For the visitor, trying to assess cruelty is made all the more difficult because we do not always know, and cannot always see, what becomes of the animals at night when all the people have gone home. Very often this is when the real process of confinement takes place. Many zoo enclosures are designed primarily for daytime occupation, with the primary design requirement of the sleeping quarters being to separate animals and keep them from physical harm until the keepers return in the morning.

Changing Public Attitudes

For years zoos have responded to accusations of cruelty by adopting a defensive attitude. They have used a 'we know best' approach, lecturing their visitors in an attempt to persuade us all to accept their definitions of what is cruel and what is not. But the tide has begun to engulf them. Public attitudes have changed faster than zoo cages. Cages that were hailed as liberating and progressive ten years ago are now seen by visitors as unacceptable. This is undoubtedly frustrating for the zoos, but if they are to survive they will have to understand that the customer is always right. They will have to learn to measure public attitudes and to keep their collections one step ahead of the moving window of public opinion. And in the end zoos ought to be prepared to accept that there may be species (like the dolphin perhaps, the orca, or the polar bear) for whom they cannot realistically recreate the fundamentals of life. If they wish to avoid accusations of cruelty then they will need to put their money where it can best be used, to help species that can best benefit with the best regard to welfare.

EVALUATING THE AUTHOR'S ARGUMENTS:

The author argues that zoos can be rated on how well they take care of animals. The authors of the previous viewpoint contend that even good zoos violate animal rights. After reading both viewpoints, do you think animal advocates should focus on improving zoos or abolishing them? Explain your answer using evidence from the viewpoints. The most common accusation levelled against zoos is one of cruelty. Is it cruel to keep animals in a zoo? Why or why not?

Chapter 3

Are Scientific Experiments on Animals Justified?

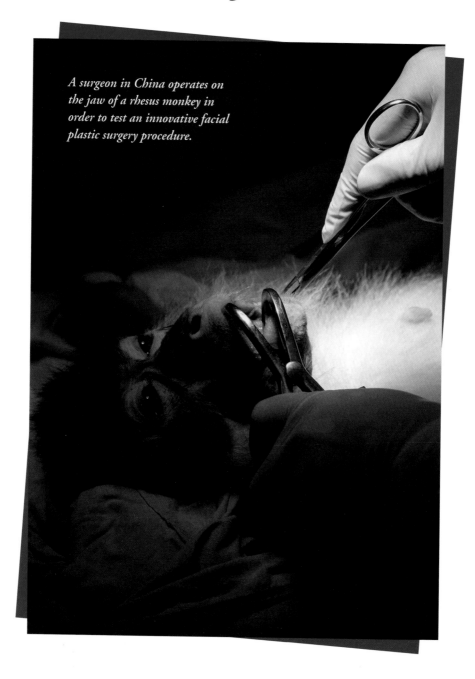

A surgeon in China operates on the jaw of a rhesus monkey in order to test an innovative facial plastic surgery procedure.

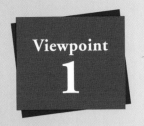

Medical Research on Apes Should Be Banned

Humane Society of the United States

"The cost of using apes in research far outweighs the benefits."

Because they are so highly developed, chimpanzees and other great apes have been at the forefront of the debate over animal experimentation. In recent years several countries, including Sweden, New Zealand, and Great Britain have banned medical research on apes. In the following viewpoint the Humane Society of the United States (HSUS) urges the United States to ban the use of apes for biomedical research. HSUS contends that apes share many mental qualities with humans, such as intelligence and capacity for emotion. These qualities make their use in experiments highly questionable. The authors also raise doubts about the scientific benefits of ape research, and note that public support for such research has been declining.

Founded in 1954, the Humane Society of the United States is one of the country's largest animal protection organizations.

The Humane Society of the United States (HSUS) is calling for an official ban on the use of nonhuman apes in biomedical research and testing in the United States. We are also calling for permanent relocation of nonhuman apes from research institutions to suitable sanctuaries as soon as possible.

Chimpanzees and Other Apes

Chimpanzees are currently the only nonhuman apes being used in biomedical research in the United States. Bonobos, gorillas, orangutans, gibbons and siamangs are currently not being used for such research. However, we are calling for a ban on research on these species in order to prevent their use in the future.

There is much debate over the use of apes in research, from an ethical and medical perspective. Are nonhuman apes scientifically "necessary" in the attempt to find cures for human disease and conditions? The physiological and behavioral similarities between human and nonhuman apes are often used as justification for conducting biomedical research on these species, yet these are the very reasons why their use poses serious ethical concerns.

Public support for the use of chimpanzees in research has been declining in recent years and this decline should be taken seriously. For example, a recent survey indicates that 54% of the public believes that it is unacceptable for chimpanzees to "undergo research which causes them to suffer for human benefit," while 65% say it is unacceptable to kill the animals for research. The results of an opinion survey conducted by the National Science Board in 2001 indicate that only 44% of all adults surveyed agreed or strongly agreed with the use of dogs and chimpanzees in scientific research (the survey did not address chimpanzees separately)—this is a 6% decrease in support compared to the 1999 results.

Ethical Concerns

Apes have many qualities that contribute to the ethical argument against their use in research. For example, apes possess complex mental abilities, including self-conception, anticipation of future events, mathematical skills, tool use and acquisition of artificial languages created by humans. They also experience a range of emotions, including depression, anxiety, pain, distress and empathy. The Boyd Group, which consists of British scientists and representatives of various organizations interested in issues regarding animal research, recently published a comprehensive document examining the use of nonhuman primates in research and testing. The document extensively discusses the various mental abilities of apes, mentioned above, and concludes: "These abilities are likely to enhance the Great Apes' capacities for suffering to such an extent that it is unethical to confine them in laboratory housing and use them in scientific procedures. A ban on the use of Great Apes in research and testing (as currently in place in the UK) is strongly supported on these grounds, as well as on grounds of conservation of species in the wild, and should be respected world-wide."[1]

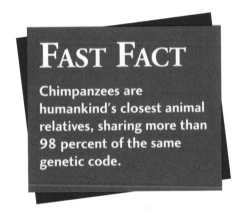

FAST FACT

Chimpanzees are humankind's closest animal relatives, sharing more than 98 percent of the same genetic code.

Medical and Scientific Concerns

An analysis conducted by the HSUS indicates that 23 institutions received $20–30 million of U.S. government funding for chimpanzee research for the year 2001. This funding was provided for research on hepatitis, HIV, cognition, genetics, neurology, drug testing, and respiratory viruses, among others. Approximately 40% of grants that pertain to chimpanzee research are for the study of various strains of hepatitis as

1. Boyd Group, *The Use of Non-Human Primates in Research and Testing.* British Psychological Society, Leicester, UK, 2002.

ANIMAL TESTING

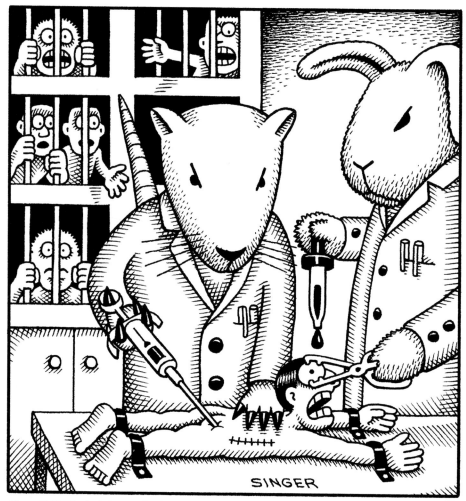

well as HIV. There was a major increase in chimpanzee breeding in the 1980s for HIV research; however, it has since been determined that chimpanzees are poor models for HIV. Despite this, significant funding for HIV research on chimpanzees continues today. It is time for these chimpanzees to be permanently relocated to a sanctuary.

Despite the striking similarities of chimpanzee and human mental abilities, these two species are different enough biologically that extrapolation of chimpanzee research results to humans is problematic. It should also be seriously considered that scientific results from any type of research conducted on apes are even further compromised as a result of their captivity-related suffering.

It Is Time to End Research on Apes

The use of apes in research, particularly chimpanzees, is declining in other areas of the world. According to a [May 2002] *Discover* article, "An Embarrassment of Chimpanzees," only the United States, Japan, Liberia, and Gabon currently use chimpanzees in biomedical research. Some countries, such as Great Britain, New Zealand, Sweden, and The Netherlands, have banned the use of great apes in research. Additionally, many of the numerous countries that do not conduct research on apes have made a conscious decision to avoid their use.

In this 1956 photograph, a monkey tests an oxygen mask at an air force research facility.

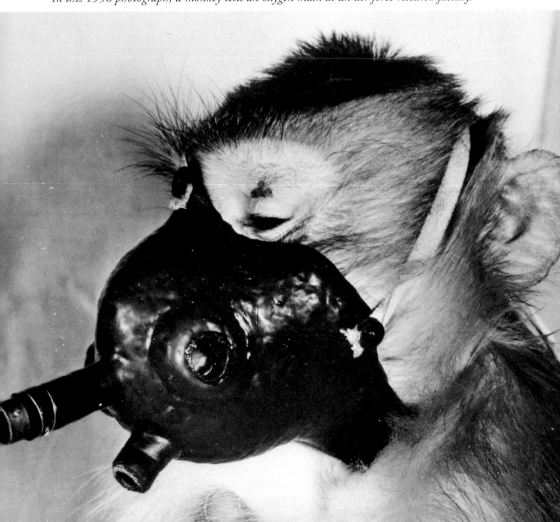

In December 2000, the United States passed the Chimpanzee Health Improvement, Maintenance and Protection (CHIMP) Act (Public Law 106-551). This legislation calls for the establishment of a national sanctuary system for chimpanzees no longer used in research. This law will not only improve living conditions for the chimpanzees, but will save the government money since sanctuary housing is significantly less expensive than laboratory housing. A recent poll commissioned by the HSUS indicates that 79% of the public supports the transfer of chimpanzees who are no longer used in research from research laboratories to sanctuaries. Passage of this legislation was a positive step, but it is time to end research on apes altogether. . . .

The United States often claims to be a leader in biomedical research, but we lag behind Europe and others in regards to research animal care, welfare and ethics. The majority of the world has decided that the cost of using apes in research far outweighs the benefits—it is time for the U.S. to come to that realization also. Ape research should be banned in the U.S. and the government should relocate chimpanzees currently housed in laboratories to appropriate sanctuaries and provide for their lifetime care.

EVALUATING THE AUTHORS' ARGUMENTS:

The Humane Society of the United States notes that America is one of only four countries that continue to use chimpanzees for research. Does this influence your opinion on whether such research is ethical? Why or why not?

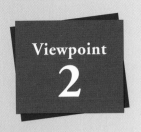

Viewpoint 2

Research on Apes Is Ethical

Wesley J. Smith

"The well-being and welfare of chimps must come second to our own."

Wesley J. Smith is an attorney and the author of many articles on the animal rights movement. In the following viewpoint he argues that the goal of saving human lives justifies medical research on apes and other animals. A ban on all animal medical research would create unnecessary human suffering by depriving people of new medicines and other medical advances, Smith contends. He believes the welfare of humans should be given a higher priority than the welfare of apes. Smith also criticizes efforts by the animal rights movement to make chimpanzees—and eventually all animals—into legal "persons" with legal rights and the same moral status as humans.

AS YOU READ, CONSIDER THE FOLLOWING QUESTIONS:

1. What is the National Institutes of Health planning to spend $24 million for, according to Smith?

2. If animals were unavailable, what might replace them as research subjects, according to the author?
3. What does the word *gestation* mean in the context of the viewpoint?

The animal-rights/liberation movement is living high on the hog these days. In the last election, for example, activists induced Florida voters to grant gestating sows a state *constitutional right* to be kept in a space large enough to turn around in. As a consequence, the two pig farms in the state that had used gestation crates to confine pregnant pigs slaughtered their herds and went out of business. This suited the animal liberationists just fine. Their ultimate goal, after all, is not merely the better treatment of pigs but an end to all animal husbandry.

A Chimp Retirement Community?

Now we learn that the National Institutes of Health (NIH) is planning to spend $24 million to build a retirement community for—no, not people—"retired" chimpanzees. The chimps in question were bred for medical research. But there are more animals than scientists need to conduct their important work to reduce human suffering, such as in researching cures for malaria.

That leaves the question of what to do with the unneeded chimps. This is an important problem. We humans have a moral obligation to treat animals properly and with humane care. Toward this end, the chimps could be given to well-managed zoos, wild-animal parks, and private primate sanctuaries. As a last and regrettable resort, if there were no option other than maintaining the animals in a cruel or inhumane manner, the chimps could be painlessly euthanized.

Instead, thanks to well-meaning but misguided congressional lawmakers back in 2000, the NIH is going to fund a cushy chimpanzee "sanctuary." Yes, you read it right. The federal government is going to put tens of millions of your taxpayer dollars into a Sun City for chimps.

In the bottomless pit that is the U.S. budget, $24 million may not seem like a lot of money. But remember, it's being taken out of funds specifically allotted for NIH, which is supposed to use its money to improve the health and welfare of people. Moreover, with the NIH budget threatened with possible new budget restrictions, this money may soon be desperately needed to fund crucial human needs. Surely research into cancer, Parkinson's disease, or AIDS should take precedence over paying for chimps to swing happily through the trees. . . .

A researcher at a New York University laboratory shares a lighthearted moment with the facility's chimpanzee subjects.

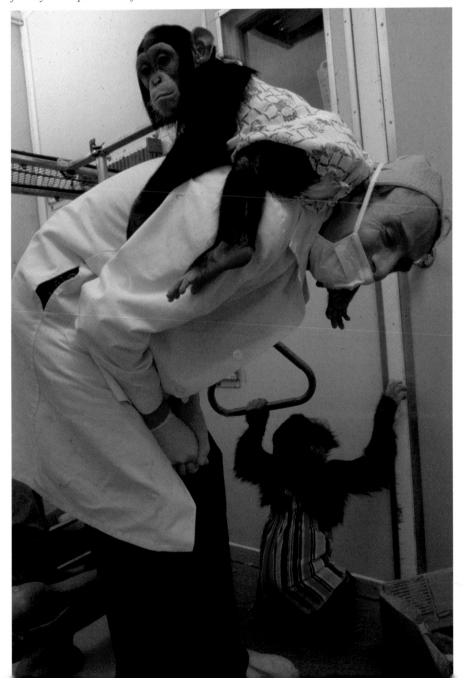

A Darker Side

There is a darker side to this story that we also should ponder. Using NIH money, as opposed to private animal-welfare philanthropy, to fund not just a shelter but a 200-acre retirement home for a few hundred chimps seems part of a wider effort by animal-rights lobbyists and liberationists to transform apes, and eventually other mammals such as pigs, dogs, elephants, and dolphins, into legal "persons."

Don't laugh. Legal clinics have already been established at some of our elite university law schools dedicated to obtaining that very objective through the courts. Indeed, advocacy seeking human/ape legal and moral equality is international in scope. The Great Ape Project, for example, explicitly states that its goal is "to include the nonhuman great apes within the community of equals by granting them the basic moral and legal protection that only human beings currently enjoy."

Making apes morally equivalent to humans would cause tremendous harm. Among the consequences: a total end to using chimps and other apes in medical research.

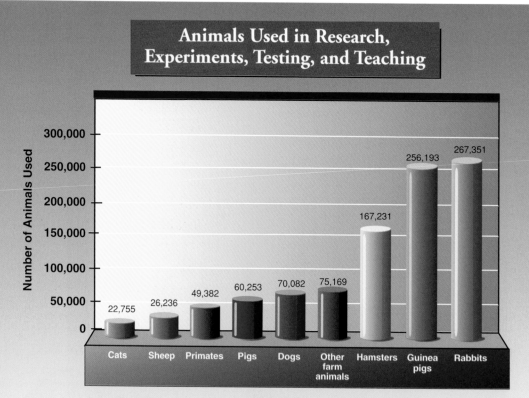

Source: U.S. Department of Agriculture, "Animal Welfare Report," 2001.

The Case for Primate Research

As unpleasant as it admittedly is, we must, on occasion, use primates as research subjects because of their intelligence and genetic closeness to human beings. Monkeys, for example, have been used in research for the treatment of paralysis caused by stroke and in AIDS research, while chimpanzees were essential to the development of the human vaccine against hepatitis B.

If these mammals became legally unavailable for this purpose, what would replace them? Actually, the question would be better phrased: "*Who* would replace them?" One possible answer was given a few years back by Princeton professor Peter Singer, the guru of the animal-liberation movement, in an interview with *Psychology Today*. When asked what alternatives he could suggest to the use of chimpanzees in medical research, he responded:

> **FAST FACT**
>
> According to the pro–animal research organization Americans for Medical Progress, scientific discoveries helped by animal research have increased the average human life span by almost twenty-eight years since 1900.

I am not comfortable with invasive research on chimps. I would ask, is there no other way? And I think there are other ways. I would say, "What about getting the consent of relatives of people in vegetative states?" If you could really confidently determine that this person will never regain consciousness, it's a lot better to use them than a chimp.

Once that ball got rolling, it wouldn't stop with the primates. Animal-rights activists seek to prevent us from using *all* animals in medical research, including mice and rats. Indeed, some animal liberationists have turned violent toward obtaining that very end, attacking laboratories, threatening researchers, and even vandalizing insurance companies that do business with medical-research facilities.

The potential harm and unnecessary human suffering that outlawing the use of animals in medical research is beyond quantifying. Think

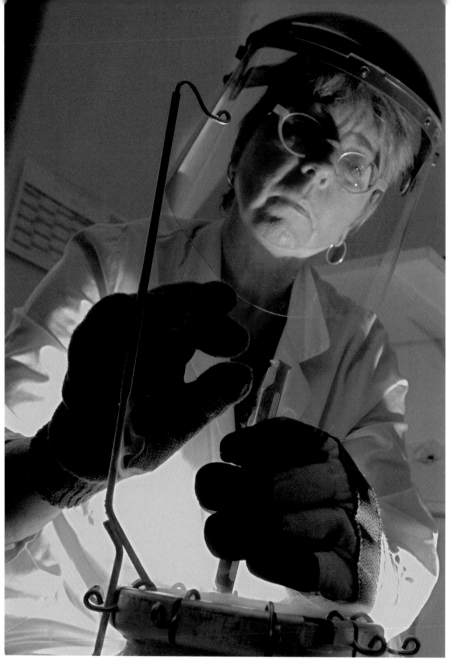

A scientist at a university in Germany works with frozen cells from apes and dogs to conduct research on a potential flu vaccine.

about it: Animals are used in stem-cell research, to test the efficacy of drugs, and in developing new surgical techniques, just to mention a few. And while some liberationists pretend that computer simulations or human tissue lines could make up the difference, in the real world that simply isn't, and may well never be, true.

Let me be clear: I recognize that chimpanzees are highly intelligent creatures that exhibit sophisticated social behavior. They have a higher capacity to suffer than do mice, rats, or birds. Hence—as empathetic, moral beings—we have a higher duty to treat them properly and humanely, both when using them as research subjects and after we no longer need them for that purpose.

Chimpanzees Are Not Persons

But as intelligent as chimpanzees are, as sophisticated as their social interactions may be, as easy as it is to anthropomorphize their lives, we must also never forget that they are animals, not persons. Toward the end of alleviating human suffering and curing human diseases, the well-being and welfare of chimps must come second to our own. That should also be true with regard to how we decide to invest our limited public-health resources. It is a disheartening sign of the times that such sentiments are now explosively controversial.

EVALUATING THE AUTHOR'S ARGUMENTS:

The author writes that humans must never forget that chimpanzees "are animals, not persons." What does he mean by this? Do you agree with this position? Explain why or why not.

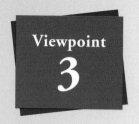

Animals Should Not Be Dissected in Biology Classes

"Classroom dissection desensitizes students to the sanctity of life and can encourage students to harm animals elsewhere."

Mercy for Animals

Each year millions of animals, ranging from worms to fetal pigs, are dissected by students in biology classes in high schools and universities. Dissection has come under increasing criticism in recent years by some educators and animal rights activists. The following viewpoint by Mercy for Animals outlines some of the arguments against this practice. The writers contend that animals used for dissection are frequently abused before they are killed. They also argue that classroom dissection desensitizes students to animal suffering. Alternatives to dissection should be pursued, the authors conclude.

Mercy for Animals is a nonprofit animal advocacy organization that conducts public education and media campaigns, animal rescues, and other activities.

AS YOU READ, CONSIDER THE FOLLOWING QUESTIONS:
1. What are six animals commonly used in dissection, according to Mercy for Animals?
2. In the authors' opinion, why is it unnecessary for most students to perform dissections?
3. What options do students have regarding dissection, according to Mercy for Animals?

D issection is the practice of cutting into and studying animals. Every year, 5.7 million animals are used in secondary and college science classes. Each animal sliced open and discarded represents not only a life lost, but also just a small part of a trail of animal abuse and environmental havoc.

Animal Victims

Frogs are the most commonly dissected animals below the university level. Other species include cats, mice, rats, worms, dogs, rabbits, fetal pigs, and fishes. The animals may come from breeding facilities which cater to institutions and businesses that use animals in experiments; they may have been caught in the wild; or they could be stolen or abandoned companion animals. An undercover investigator at one of the nation's largest suppliers of animals for dissection was told by his supervisor that some of the cats killed there were companion animals who had "escaped" from their homes. Slaughterhouses and pet stores also sell animals and animal parts to biological supply houses.

Investigators documented cases of animals being removed from gas chambers and injected with formaldehyde without first being checked for vital signs (a violation of the Animal Welfare Act). (Formaldehyde is a severely irritating caustic substance which causes

> **FAST FACT**
>
> In some medical schools, first-year students operate on living dogs to practice surgery and learn anatomy. However, many schools, including Harvard, Yale, and Stanford, have abolished dog labs.

a painful death.) Investigators videotaped cats and rats struggling during infusion and employees spitting on the animals.

Frogs are captured in the wild to stock breeding ponds because populations die out if not replenished. A completely independent frog colony has never survived long without the introduction of "outside" frogs.

In their natural habitat, frogs consume large numbers of insects responsible for crop destruction and the spread of disease. In the years preceding India's ban on the frog trade, that country was earning $10 million a year from frog exports, but spending $100 million to import chemical pesticides to fight insect infestations. In addition, economic losses in agricultural produce were heavy. Today, Bangladesh is the main Asian market for frogs, and in the United States, scientists have noted severe declines in frog and toad populations that they blame on the capture of these animals for food and experiments, as well as on causes of general environmental decline such as the use of pesticides and habitat destruction.

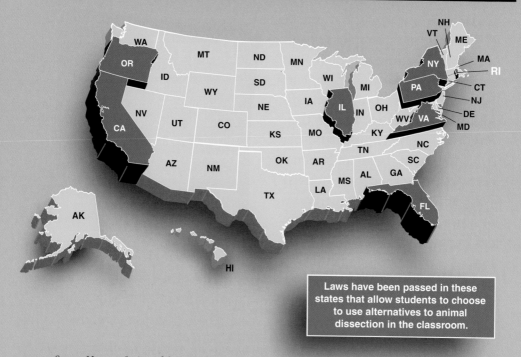

States with Animal Dissection Choice Laws for Students

Laws have been passed in these states that allow students to choose to use alternatives to animal dissection in the classroom.

Source: Humane Society of the United States, www.hsus.org/dissection_laws.

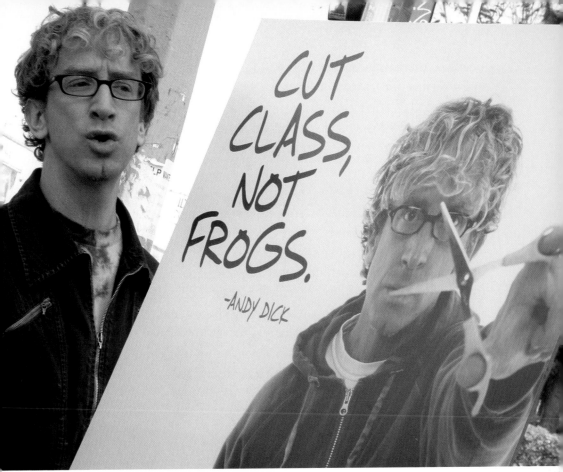

Comedian and actor Andy Dick urges students at a high school in Hollywood not to participate in classroom dissection.

Dissection Is Not Educational

Classroom dissection desensitizes students to the sanctity of life and can encourage students to harm animals elsewhere, perhaps in their own backyard. In fact, serial killer Jeffrey Dahmer attributed his fascination with murder and mutilation to classroom dissections. In the last interview before his death, televised on *Dateline NBC,* Dahmer stated, "In 9th grade, in biology class, we had the usual dissection of fetal pigs, and I took the remains of that [pig] home and kept the skeleton of it, and I just started branching out to dogs, cats." According to Dahmer, he enjoyed the excitement and power he experienced when cutting up animals and fantasized about cutting up a human body.

Students with little or no interest in pursuing a career in science certainly don't need to see actual organs to understand basic physiology, and students who are planning on pursuing a career in biology or medicine would do better to study humans in a controlled, supervised setting, or to study human cadavers or some of the sophisticated alternatives, such as computer models. Those who are rightfully disturbed by the prospect of cutting up animals will be too preoccupied by their concerns to learn anything of value during the dissection.

Students Can Take a Stand

More and more students are taking a stand against dissection before it happens in their classes, from the elementary school level on up to veterinary and medical school. In 1987, Jenifer Graham objected to dissection and was threatened with a lower grade. Jenifer went to court to plead her case and later testified before the California legislature, which responded by passing a law giving students in the state the right not to dissect. . . . Since Jenifer's case, thousands of students have opted to study biology in humane ways, and many schools have accepted the students' right to violence-free education.

EVALUATING THE AUTHORS' ARGUMENTS:

Mercy for Animals cites the case of Jeffrey Dahmer, a notorious serial killer who cut apart and ate his victims. They argue that his penchant for killing was caused in part by his experience with classroom dissections. Do you think it is reasonable to use Dahmer as an example of why animals should not be dissected? Explain your answer.

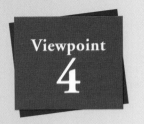

Viewpoint

4

Animal Dissection Can Be a Valuable Teaching Tool

John Richard Schrock

In recent years dissection of animals for biology classes has been questioned. In the following viewpoint biology professor John Richard Schrock argues that dissection can provide an important hands-on learning experience for students that cannot be replicated with alternative teaching methods such as computer models and simulations. Through dissection, Schrock asserts, students can better learn about animal anatomy, laboratory techniques, and other important topics. Dissection may also inspire students to become surgeons or medical professionals.

Schrock chairs the biology department at Emporia State University in Kansas. This viewpoint is excerpted from the "Ask an Expert" feature in the newsletter for the National Association of Biology Teachers.

"Dissection is interesting and motivating."

John Richard Schrock, "How Do You Make Dissection Exciting?" *News & Views,* January 2005. Copyright © 2005 by the National Association of Biology Teachers. Reproduced by permission.

AS YOU READ, CONSIDER THE FOLLOWING QUESTIONS:
1. Why does the author believe it is important to learn about variation in biology?
2. Why is it important for students to overcome being squeamish about the messy aspects of dissection, according to the author?
3. What does *palpation* mean in the context of this viewpoint?

*D*ear Expert: How do I get my students interested in dissection? Without curiosity, dissection feels like busy work. I want to make this experience more than an exercise in memorizing body parts.

Dissection is interesting and motivating for the same reason that all real labwork and fieldwork is intrinsically interesting and motivating:

The most meaningful definition of an organism is the actual organism, not an abstraction. Many parents will relate that the only thing they remember from a biology class decades ago is a frog dissection, testimony to the lasting memory of multisensory, hands-on experiences.

The Limits of Computer Simulations

Real material is truly interactive; "interaction" with a computer keyboard is a trivial use of the term, and completely unrelated to the genuine interaction of touching an earthworm crop and gizzard, petting a gerbil, or holding a harmless snake.

Real material is test-truthful. Texts and simulations present perfect examples, from anatomy to 3-to-1 hybrid crosses. Teachers of dissection labs spot anomalies and call students over to see the cat with three carotid arteries or four kidneys or, rarely, left-right reversal. Variation in biology is an important lesson for future patients who otherwise might expect perfection and predictability in medicine.

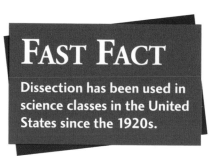

FAST FACT

Dissection has been used in science classes in the United States since the 1920s.

Learning to observe involves practice tracing pathways, detecting textures, and combining reasoning with dissection skills. The organs of a fish, unlike a diagram, are not color-coded; tracing the digestive system requires probing. The small, delicate anatomy of a grasshopper is too advanced for beginners, but becomes easy after a student develops skills. . . .

Palpation is a valuable diagnostic skill. The crop and gizzard of the earthworm are distinguished more by feel than appearance. Only a few students will become physicians who will use palpation to assess the liver or identify organs in a pelvic or prostate exam, but all students will become patients who need to understand and be comfortable with palpation.

High school students in Chandler, Arizona, dissect pigs in their advanced biology class.

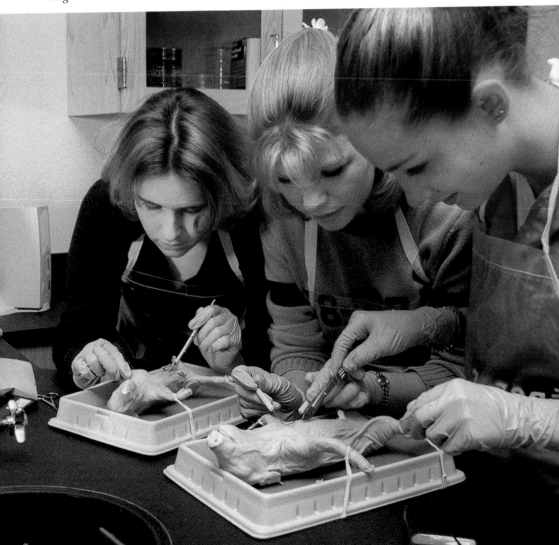

Top Eight Animals Teachers Use in Classroom Dissection

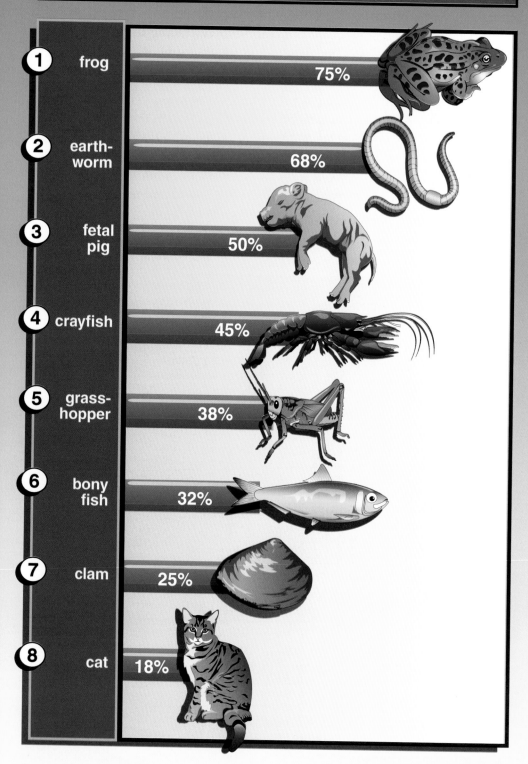

1. frog — 75%
2. earthworm — 68%
3. fetal pig — 50%
4. crayfish — 45%
5. grasshopper — 38%
6. bony fish — 32%
7. clam — 25%
8. cat — 18%

Source: Information compiled from a survey of five thousand biology teachers who reported using dissection; Humane Society of the United States, www.hsus.org, 2004.

Overcoming Squeamishness

Being squeamish about blood, feces, or cutting of tissue is a handicap. Normalization is necessary for surgeons and nurses to be able to function. Parents have to apply bandages and diaper babies.

Indeed, some students will eventually become surgeons and health-care professionals. Many of them have traced their initial interest to these very lab experiences. We cannot accurately predict which students will become fascinated and pursue a health career or join the science pipeline.

Real labwork has real consequences. When students have successfully mastered a procedure or technique, they know they can really do it in the real world. When they click through a simulation, they have merely completed an artificial game. . . .

Creating New Understanding

After our pre-service teachers visited an upper elementary class and helped small groups of students each dissect a cow eyeball with care and respect, one student wrote, "When I've been to science workshops before, all those names and long words haven't meant a thing. But now I understand."

EVALUATING THE AUTHORS' ARGUMENTS:

The author of this viewpoint discusses what he considers to be important benefits of exposing students to animal dissection. The authors of the previous viewpoint outline what they think are the drawbacks of the practice. After reading both viewpoints, what is your opinion of animal dissection? Cite from the texts to support your argument.

Pet Cloning Harms Animals

Jennifer Fearing

> *"The 'promise' of pet cloning isn't humane —to either the animals or the humans involved."*

Some of the most controversial animal research involves cloning. In August 2005 researchers in South Korea successfully cloned a dog, while researchers in the United States have cloned cats. Following these developments, some commercial enterprises have been established to help pet owners clone their favorite animal. Jennifer Fearing writes in the following viewpoint that pet cloning is unethical and should be discouraged. She argues that the cloning procedure involves cruelty to animals and their offspring, most of which do not survive the process. Fearing also argues that pet owners should not spend thousands of dollars to replace their pet with a clone when they could go to their local animal shelter and adopt another cat or dog who needs a home.

Jennifer Fearing is cofounder of Californians Against Pet Cloning. She has worked to pass legislation against animal cloning.

Amid all the fanfare and smiling portraits heralding the birth of Snuppy, the world's first cloned dog, there is a dark and unsettling side to animal cloning that even the scientists involved readily admit, but which gets far less attention than it deserves.

Cloning Has Low Success Rates

Glossed over with language like "inefficiency" and "high failure rates," scientists roundly agree that animal cloning leaves a lot to be desired. Managing large numbers of animals over long periods of time to yield "success rates" of between 0.5 percent and 4 percent isn't anyone's idea of a good investment. At the low end of this range, this means that it can take more than 200 animals surgically impregnated to yield a single clone birth.

Along the way, in each of these grand experiments, these 200 animals are housed in laboratories and subjected to multiple invasive surgeries, to say nothing of the very few they actually give birth to—clones whose lives are often short and painful.

> **FAST FACT**
>
> The Humane Society estimates that 6 to 8 million dogs and cats are placed in animal shelters each year, and 3 to 4 million animals are euthanized annually.

According to their findings published in the journal *Nature* last week [August 2005], the scientists involved in Snuppy's production surgically implanted 123 surrogate dogs with embryos that resulted in only three pregnancies, two deliveries and one puppy surviving the first month of life. The only other viable puppy succumbed to pneumonia

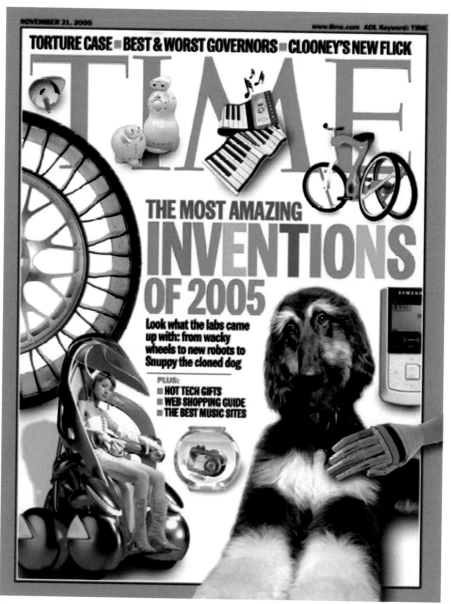

Snuppy, the world's first cloned dog, was featured on the cover of the November 13, 2005, edition of Time *magazine.*

at 22 days, after suffering respiratory distress throughout his short life in the laboratory.

The False Promise of Pet Cloning
And while some see animal cloning as an opportunity—albeit grotesquely inefficient and arguably immoral—to advance animal

or human health, others are engaged in the effort strictly as a for-profit venture to reproduce people's pets. The wholly unregulated company that sold the cat Little Nicky as a clone for $50,000 in December [2004] is aggressively marketing its gene-banking services to veterinarians and to pet lovers across the country through direct mail and ambitious public-relations strategies. Despite having produced only a handful of cat clones and no dogs, this company, based in Sausalito, will happily take your $1,395 (plus $150 a year in storage fees) along with Fido's or Fluffy's DNA, on the off chance you can one day afford to pay the remaining $30,000 to order up your clone. All this while, millions of healthy and adoptable cats and dogs die every year only because there are not enough homes.

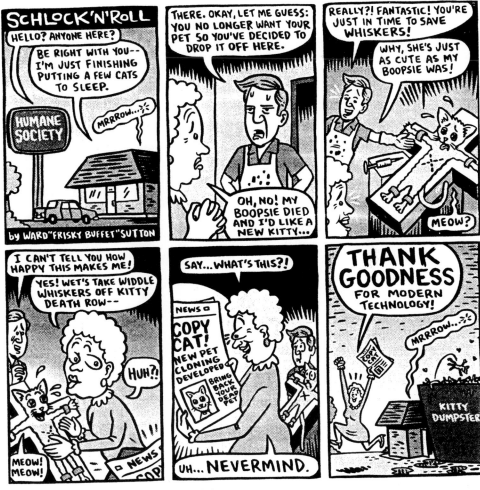

Sutton. © by Ward Sutton. Reproduced by permission.

I'll admit to being especially fond of animals, but I don't know any pet lover who would willingly comply with a process that caused the pain and suffering of hundreds of animals to clone his or her favorite pet. Once people really understand that the odds are better than not that the clone will not act and possibly not even look like the animal they hope to replace, most are turned off. They're among more than 80 percent of the American public who are opposed to pet cloning, according to a poll commissioned by the American Anti-Vivisection Society. Those who fall for cloning's false promise are being misled, blinded by the grief of losing their beloved companion, or are more interested in vanity and novelty than they are in what it means to be a companion in the first place.

Some animal welfare advocates argue that instead of cloning pets, people should adopt animals from shelters.

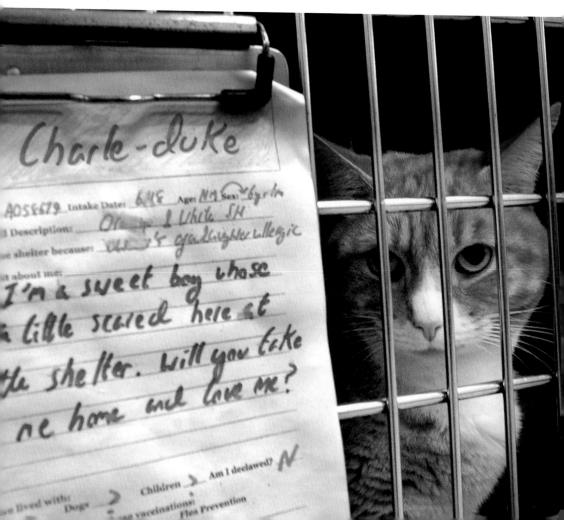

Pet Cloning Should Be Banned

It is out of these concerns that we formed Californians Against Pet Cloning [in 2004] and introduced Assembly Bill 1428 to ban the retail sale of cloned and genetically modified pets. While the bill got held up in committee this [2004–2005] session, we will continue to press policymakers to address the serious ethical, consumer protection and animal-welfare concerns that are raised by for-profit and trivial animal experimentation.

Don't be fooled by the cute photos. For every one of those kittens and puppies that they bring out into the light, there are hundreds more who suffered to make that photo op possible. The "promise" of pet cloning isn't humane—to either the animals or the humans involved. It is a consumer fraud and an animal welfare atrocity.

EVALUATING THE AUTHOR'S ARGUMENTS:

Fearing argues that real animal and pet lovers will not support pet cloning. After reading the viewpoint, do you agree or disagree? What arguments to you find the most or least convincing?

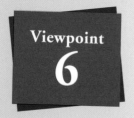

Pet Cloning Does Not Harm Animals

Autumn Fiester

"If animal welfare worries are truly the motivation for critiquing cat cloning, then the concern is misplaced."

Autumn Fiester is head of graduate studies at the Center for Bioethics at the University of Pennsylvania. She has written several articles on the morality of animal cloning. In the following viewpoint she argues that pet cloning does not pose serious ethical issues. The science of cloning is improving, she writes, and worries about the health and survival of clones will not be an issue in the future. She also argues that there is little need to worry about the welfare of cloned pets because they will be loved and well cared for. Fiester concludes that the potential to create animals that are combinations of different species is far more worrisome than cloning pets.

AS YOU READ, CONSIDER THE FOLLOWING QUESTIONS:

1. How much did one pet owner pay for a clone of a pet cat, according to Fiester?

2. What response does the author make to the argument that spending money to clone a pet is irresponsible when unwanted pets are readily available in animal shelters?
3. What does the word *euthanized* mean in the context of the viewpoint?

Pet cloning is now officially a commercial enterprise. For the price of $50,000, a Texas woman commissioned a clone of her beloved cat "Nicky," and today [January 2005] she is the proud owner of that cat's genetic twin, aka "Little Nicky." The creation and sale of Little Nicky has sparked intense criticism from bioethicists across the country, who label the pet cloning venture everything from "frivolous" to "reprehensible." But in the unregulated land of animal biotechnology, cloning pets for devout animal lovers seems like the least of our animal welfare problems.

Pet Cloning Is Ethical

The most serious concern critics raise about pet cloning is the suffering of the clones, which are sometimes born with health problems or don't survive past infancy. But cloning science is advancing so rapidly that the survival rates and general health of clones are beginning to mirror animals naturally conceived. So this will soon be a non-starter.

What criticisms remain? The most common complaint is that it's wrong to spend $50,000 to clone a pet when millions of unwanted animals are euthanized in shelters each year. This is an odd argument for a lot of reasons. First, there's nothing different about this use of money and any other luxury purchase—the money could always be better spent if put towards noble causes like fighting world hunger or curing AIDS. This fact doesn't

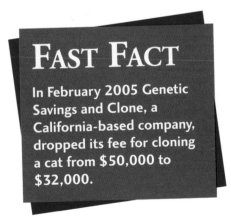

FAST FACT

In February 2005 Genetic Savings and Clone, a California-based company, dropped its fee for cloning a cat from $50,000 to $32,000.

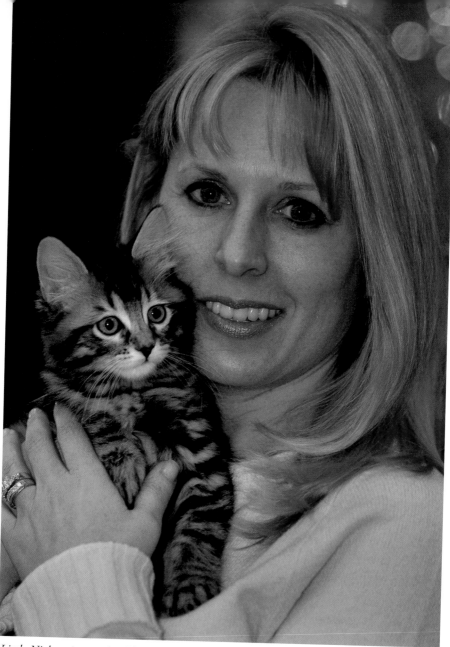

Little Nicky, nine weeks old, is held by his owner, who paid $50,000 to have him cloned from her deceased cat.

make pet cloning any different ethically than boat-buying. And why would a person who was devoted to a particular animal be more obligated than the rest of us to save others of that species—let alone members of other species? Finally, the criticism misses the point of pet cloning: pet owners don't want just any old cat.

They see their original animal as a unique being, not one that's exchangeable. They spend the money on cloning because the closest they can come to getting that particular animal back is having the identical twin of their beloved pet.

"Frankenpets" Are the Real Worry

If animal welfare worries are truly the motivation for critiquing cat cloning, then the concern is misplaced. Little Nicky, and other clones like him, will thrive and end up being some of the most pampered pets in America. What ought to really worry us is an animal biotechnology industry that is wholly unregulated and may have more imagination than good sense. The real "Frankenpets" are just around the corner: transgenic animals and chimeras that will be conglomerations of different species spliced together. The Glofish and Alba the Green Bunny are just the first in a long line. These animals will make run-of-the-mill cat cloning seem dull. But how much will these strange animals suffer? How will these animals impact other animals or the ecosystem? If we are going to put animal cloning on our moral agenda, it's not pet cloning that we should worry about.

EVALUATING THE AUTHORS' ARGUMENTS:

Fiester argues that animal welfare worries about pet cloning are misplaced because the animals to be cloned will be truly pampered and loved. Do you believe this is an adequate response to the concerns raised by Fearing in the opposing viewpoint? Why or why not?

Glossary

animal welfare: The protection of the health and well-being of animals.

Animal Welfare Act: U.S. law passed in 1966 that sets the standards for the handling, housing, feeding, and caring of animals in laboratories, zoos, circuses, and pet stores.

antivivisectionist: A person who is opposed to operating on or experimenting with living animals.

biomedical: Refers to a combination of medical, biological, and physical sciences. Biomedical research often studies how humans or animals cope with stressful situations, such as injury or illness.

cruelty-free products: Products that have not been tested on animals.

dissection: Cutting up animal or human bodies for scientific research.

free-range farms: Farms where animals are given relative freedom to roam and forage instead of being restricted to cages.

fur farms: Farms where fur-bearing animals, such as mink, are raised for the use of their pelts.

game: Animals and birds that are usually hunted, such as deer.

humane: Kind, tender, merciful, or considerate.

livestock: Farm animals, such as horses, cattle, and pigs.

vegan: A person who does not eat any form of meat, including beef, pork, chicken, and fish, or any animal product, including cheese, milk, eggs, and sometimes honey.

vegetarian: A person who does not eat any form of meat, including beef, pork, fish, and chicken.

vivisection: Operating or experimenting on living animals to observe biological processes.

Facts About Animal Rights

Editor's Note: These facts can be used in reports or papers to reinforce or add credibility when making important points or claims.

Animals and Food

- Americans consume 270 pounds (122.5kg) of beef per person every year.
- According to the American Heart Association, 60 million Americans suffer from coronary heart disease in part because they eat meat.
- Cattle raised for beef are typically slaughtered when they are 15 to 20 months old. If not slaughtered, the lifespan of cattle averages 20 to 25 years.
- Cows produce 86 percent of the world's milk. Other animals milked for human use include water buffalo, llamas, goats, sheep, horses, and reindeer.
- On average, Americans consume about three 8-ounce (236.7ml) glasses of milk a day.
- Over 260 million turkeys were slaughtered for food in 2003 in the United States, most at about fourteen to eighteen weeks of age.
- Poultry accounts for 95 percent of animals killed for food in the United States.
- In some chicken farm operations, chickens have their beaks removed to prevent them from pecking each other to death.

Animals and Research

- The U.S. Department of Agriculture stated in its 2004 *Animal Care Report* that 64,932 dogs, 54,998 primates, and 23,640 cats were used for medical research.
- Ninety-five percent of animals bred for medical research in the United States are mice and rats.
- The medical advances obtained with the help of animal experimentation include: open-heart surgery, the development of anthrax, polio,

and rabies vaccines; the discovery of insulin; and gene transfer treatment for cystic fibrosis.

- Animal rights activists oppose the following scientific tests:

Draize test. A test substance placed in the eyes of rabbits or other animals; the resulting eye damage is observed. Used to predict if substance will cause skin irritation in humans.

Skin irritancy test. The test substance is applied to shaved areas of an animal's skin to determine sensitivity.

Lethal Dose 50 Test. Also called the acute toxicity test. Animals are given a substance until 50 percent of them have been killed; the remaining animals are killed and autopsied to see how the substance affected their organs and tissues.

Source: Animal Protection Institute (www.api4animals.com).

Animals and the Law

- The federal Humane Slaughter Act, passed in 1958 and amended in 1978, requires that animals be rendered insensible to pain before they are slaughtered.

- Chicken and other birds are not covered by the Humane Slaughter Act.

- The Animal Welfare Act (AWA), passed in 1966 and amended in 2002, regulates the handling of warm-blooded animals used in research, bred for commercial sale, exhibited to the public, or commercially transported. The act requires animals to be treated with minimum standards of care.

- The AWA does not apply to cold-blooded animals such as fish and reptiles. It also does not apply to farm animals used for food or fiber. It does apply to farm animals being used for biomedical research.

Historical Landmarks of the Animal Rights and Welfare Movements

1641 Massachusetts Bay Colony passes a law stating that "No man shall exercise any Tyranny or Cruelty towards any creature which is usually kept for man's use."

1824 The Society for the Prevention of Cruelty to Animals (later called the Royal Society of Prevention of Cruelty to Animals) is formed in England.

1835 Massachusetts becomes the first state to enact animal anticruelty statutes.

1866 The American Society for the Prevention of Cruelty to Animals is founded with the intent of "promoting humane principles, preventing cruelty, and alleviating pain, fear and suffering in all animals."

1907 All American states adopt statutes banning cruelty to animals.

1972 The Animal Liberation Front is founded in England. The radical group becomes notorious for its various "direct action" campaigns ranging from vandalism to break-ins at animal research laboratories.

1979 Animal rights and welfare activists succeed in repealing the Metcalf-Hatch Act, a New York state law that had permitted scientists to seize and utilize unclaimed animals from shelters for use in medical experiments.

1980 People for the Ethical Treatment of Animals (PETA) is founded.

1996 The first world congress on alternatives to animal experimentation is held in the Netherlands.

American Anti-Vivisection Society (AAVS)
801 Old York Rd., Suite 204, Jenkintown, PA 19046-1685
(215) 887-0816
e-mail: aavs@aavs.org
Web site: www.aavs.org

AAVS opposes all types of experiments on living animals and sponsors research on alternatives to these methods.

American Meat Institute (AMI)
1700 N. Moore St., Suite 1600, Arlington, VA 22209
(703) 841-2400
Web site: www.meatami.com
Founded in 1906, the AMI is a membership trade organization that represents the interests of the meat and poultry industries. The AMI Web site posts news releases, fact sheets, info kits, and visual aids relating to animal welfare.

Americans for Medical Progress
908 King St., Suite 201, Alexandria, VA 22314-3067
(703) 836-9595
Web site: www.ampef.org

The organization's mission is to promote public understanding of and support for the appropriate role of animals in biomedical research.

American Society for the Prevention of Cruelty to Animals (ASPCA)
424 E. Ninety-second St., New York, NY 10128-6804
(212) 876-7700
Web site: www.aspca.org

The ASPCA promotes appreciation for and humane treatment of animals and works for the passage of legislation that strengthens existing animal protection laws.

American Zoo and Aquarium Association (AZA)
8403 Colesville Rd., Suite 710, Silver Spring, MD 20910-3314
(301) 562-0777
Web site: www.aza.org

AZA represents over two hundred zoos and aquariums in North America. The association provides information on captive breeding of endangered species, conservation education, natural history, and wildlife legislation.

Animal Alliance of Canada
221 Broadview Ave., Suite 101, Toronto, ON M4M 2G3 Canada
(416) 462-9541
e-mail: info@animalalliance.ca
Web site: www.animalalliance.ca

The Animal Alliance of Canada is an animal rights advocacy and education group. It investigates the conditions under which millions of animals live and publishes its findings in fact sheets and in its *Take Action* newsletter.

Animal Legal Defense Fund (ALDF)
127 Fourth St., Petaluma, CA 94952-3005
(707) 769-7771
e-mail: info@aldf.org
Web site: www.aldf.org

ALDF is an organization of attorneys and law students who promote animal rights and protect the lives and interests of animals through the use of their legal skills.

Foundation for Biomedical Research (FBR)
818 Connecticut Ave. NW, Suite 900, Washington, DC 20006
(202) 457-0654
Web site: www.fbresearch.org

FBR provides information and educational programs about what it sees as the necessary and important role of laboratory animals in biomedical research and testing. It produces position papers, fact sheets, and classroom materials on animal testing.

Fund for Animals
200 W. Fifty-seventh St., New York, NY 10019
(212) 246-2096
e-mail: fundinfo@fund.org
Web site: www.fund.org

The Fund for Animals publicizes animal protection issues, facilitates the passage of pro-animal legislation, and helps to stave off bills that would allow animals to be exploited or harmed.

The Great Ape Project (GAP)
PO Box 19492, Portland, OR 97280-0492
(503) 222-5755
Web site: www.greatapeproject.org

GAP, an international organization, argues that due to their humanlike mental capacities and emotions, apes deserve the same basic moral and legal rights as people.

Humane Society of the United States (HSUS)
2100 L St. NW, Washington, DC 20037
(202) 452-1100
Web site: www.hsus.org

HSUS promotes responsible pet ownership and the elimination of cruelty to animals in hunting, trapping, and other areas.

Institute for Animal Rights Law
6 Overlook Rd., Santa Fe, NM 87505
Web site: www.instituteforanimalrightslaw.org

Institute for Animal Rights Law provides legal information, analysis, and guidance for the animal rights and animal welfare movements. Its Web site offers model statutes, federal animal protection statutes, and articles pertaining to animal rights law.

Medical Research Modernization Committee (MRMC)
PO Box 20971, Cleveland, OH 44120
(216) 283-6702
Web site: www.mrmcmed.org/main.html

The MRMC is a national health advocacy group composed of physicians, scientists, and other health care professionals who evaluate benefits, risks, and costs of medical research methods and technologies. It opposes research on animals.

National Animal Interest Alliance (NAIA)
PO Box 66579, Portland, OR 97266
(503) 761-1139
Web site: www.naiaonline.org

NAIA represents a broad spectrum of animal owners, including farmers, scientists, and pet owners. It supports legal protections, but not legal rights, for animals.

People for the Ethical Treatment of Animals (PETA)
501 Front St., Norfolk, VA 23510
(757) 622-PETA (7382)
e-mail: peta@norfolk.infi.net
Web site: www.peta.org

PETA works to establish and protect the rights of animals and focuses primarily on research laboratories, the fur trade, the entertainment industry, and factory farms. It publishes the children's magazine *Animal Times, Grrr!*

Performing Animals Welfare Society (PAWS)
PO Box 840, Galt, CA 95632
(209) 745-2606
Web site: www.pawsweb.org

Founded in 1985, PAWS provides sanctuary to abandoned and abused performing animals from circuses, zoos, rodeos, and other entertainment venues.

Zoocheck Canada
2646 St. Clair Ave. East, Toronto, ON M4B 3M1 Canada
(416) 285-1744
e-mail: zoocheck@zoocheck.com
Web site: www.zoocheck.com

Zoocheck Canada aims to protect animal welfare through investigation, research, campaigns, and legal actions. Many of the news articles and reports on its Web site discuss animal welfare across the globe.

For Further Reading

Books

Cavalieri, Paola, *The Animal Question: Why Nonhuman Animals Deserve Human Rights*. New York: Oxford University Press, 2001. Examines the philosophical reasoning why animals have rights.

Cohen, Carl, and Tom Regan, *The Animal Rights Debate*. Lanhan, MD: Rowman & Littlefield, 2001. Two philosophers with opposing views on whether animals have rights discuss and defend their beliefs.

Currie-McGhee, Leanne K., *Animal Rights*. San Diego: Lucent, 2005. An informative and readable overview that examines how animals are used as food and for science and entertainment and covers both sides of the animal rights debate.

Francione, Gary L., *Introduction to Animal Rights: Your Child or Your Dog?* Philadelphia: Temple University Press, 2000. A law professor makes the argument for animal rights.

Gaughen, Shasta, ed., *Animal Rights: Contemporary Issues Companion*. San Diego: Greenhaven, 2005. An anthology of articles on animal rights issues including vegetarianism and animal experimentation.

Greek, C. Ray, and Jean Swingle Greek, *Sacred Cows and Golden Geese: The Human Cost of Experiments on Animals*. New York: Continuum International, 2000. Argues that the use of animals in experiments is unnecessary and can even produce inaccurate results.

Jones, Barbara, *Animal Rights*. Austin, TX: Raintree SteckVaughn, 1999. A readable exploration of animal rights issues.

Kistler, John M., *People Promoting and People Opposing Animal Rights: In Their Own Words*. Westport, CT: Greenwood, 2002. A collection of profiles of people actively involved in animal rights and animal welfare movements.

Machan, Tibor R., *Putting Humans First: Why We Are Nature's Favorite*. Lanham, MD: Rowman & Littlefield, 2004. The author defends human exploitation of animals and rebuts the notion that nonhuman animals have rights.

Newkirk, Ingrid, *You Can Save the Animals: 251 Simple Ways to Stop Animal Cruelty*. Rocklin, CA: Prima, 1999. The cofounder of the organization People for the Ethical Treatment of Animals (PETA) describes ways people can help protect animals from human cruelty and exploitation.

Paul, Ellen Frankel, and Jeffrey Paul, eds., *Why Animal Experimentation Matters: The Use of Animals in Medical Research*. New Brunswick, NJ: Transaction, 2001. An anthology of essays, most of which defend the practice of animal experimentation.

Regan, Tom, *Defending Animal Rights*. Urbana: University of Illinois Press, 2001. A collection of speeches and writings from one of the foremost philosophers of animal rights.

Scully, Matthew, *Dominion: The Power of Man, the Suffering of Animals, and the Call to Mercy*. New York: St. Martin's, 2002. The writer, a former speechwriter to President George W. Bush, criticizes some of the rhetoric of the animal rights movement but argues that humans have the responsibility to treat animals humanely.

Singer, Pete, ed., *In Defense of Animals: The Second Wave*. Oxford, UK: Blackwell, 2005. The author of the influential 1975 book *Animal Liberation* assesses the state of the animal rights movement in this anthology of articles.

Sunstein, Cass R., and Martha C. Nussbaum, eds., *Animal Rights: Current Debates and New Directions*. New York: Oxford University Press, 2004. An anthology featuring articles by both proponents and opponents of animal rights.

Treanor, Nick, ed., *The History of Issues: Animal Rights*. San Diego: Greenhaven, 2005. A collection of historical and recent writings on animal rights topics.

Wise, Stephen M., *Drawing the Line: Science and the Case for Animal Rights*. Cambridge, MA: Perseus, 2002. The author, a lawyer and animal rights advocate, compares the mental abilities of various animals, including a chimpanzee, a parrot, and a dolphin, along with his four-year-old son, and concludes that some animals should be recognized as legal persons.

Workman, Dave, *PETA Files: The Dark Side of the Animal Rights Movement*. Bellevue, WA: Merril, 2003. An outdoor writer and investigative journalist argues that animal rights activists are implicated in acts of vandalism and violence.

Periodicals

Atlantic Monthly, "Animal Testing," December 2003.

Best, Stephen, "Chewing on the Rights vs. Welfare Debate: Do Corporate Reforms Delay Animal Liberation?" *Animals' Agenda*, March/April 2002.

Bok, Hilary, "Cloning Companion Animals Is Wrong," *Journal of Applied Animal Welfare Science*, 2002.

Brown, Heidi, "Beware of People," *Forbes*, July 26, 2004.

Clarke, Jeremy, "Animals Don't Have Human Rights," *Spectator*, January 2, 2005.

Cohen, Julie, "Monkey Puzzles (Basic Legal Rights for Animals)," *Geographical*, May 2000.

Current Events, "Fur Flies over Flier: Does PETA Unfairly Target Teens?" November 5, 2004.

———, "Should You Cut That Frog? A Cut-Throat Debate over Dissection," November 1, 2002.

Dreifus, Claudia, "A Courtroom Champion for 4-Legged Creatures," *New York Times*, October 1, 2002.

Economist, "Playing Terrorists: Animal Rights Extremism," April 17, 2004.

Festing, Simon, and Ray Greek, "Animal Research: Necessary Evil . . . or Both?" *Economist*, November 2003.

Francione, Gary L., "Animals and Us: Our Hypocrisy," *New Scientist*, June 4, 2005.

Freedman, Jeffery M., "Why I Am a Vegan," *Tikkun*, May/June 2003.

Keating, Susan Katz, "Animal Rights & Wrongs," *American Legion*, November 2003.

Lancet, "Animal Research Is a Source of Human Compassion, Not Shame," September 4, 2004.

Madigan, Nick, "Enlisting Law Schools in Campaign for Animals," *New York Times*, November 27, 2004.

Motavalli, Jim, "Across the Great Divide: Environmentalists and Animal Rights Activists Battle over Vegetarianism," *E Magazine*, January/February 2002.

Nordlinger, Jay, "PETA vs. KFC: A Dirty War Against the Colonel," *National Review*, December 22, 2003.

Righton, Barbara, "All the Sad Horses," *Macleans*, February 10, 2003.

Sapontzis, S.F., "Unethical Considerations: Probing Animal Research," *AV Magazine*, Spring 2002.

Satchell, Michael, "Terrorize People, Save Animals," *U.S. News & World Report*, April 8, 2002.

Schamberg, Kirsten, and Tim Jones, "Ground Zero of Labs vs. Animal Rights Activists," *Chicago Tribune*, June 13, 2005.

Smith, Wesley J., "Dying for Liberation: Why Is PETA Killing Animals?" *National Review*, July 13, 2005.

Specter, Michael, "The Extremist," *New Yorker*, April 14, 2003.

Web Sites

All-Creatures.org (www.all-creatures.org). A Web resource dedicated to cruelty-free living through a vegetarian-vegan lifestyle according to Judeo-Christian ethics. It contains thousands of text documents on animals and animal rights.

Animalrights.net (www.animalrights.net). This Web site features information and discussion forums critical of the animal rights movement. It supports the use of animals in research, food, fur, and many other common uses.

Animal Rights Law Project (www.animal-law.org). A Web site created by law professors and students at Rutgers University, the first law school in the United States to teach animal rights as part of its regular curriculum. It includes essays on animal rights, state and federal animal laws and regulations, and selected documents from legal actions involving animal abuse.

AnimalScam.com (www.animalscam.com). AnimalScam.com, a project of the nonprofit organization Center for Consumer Freedom, refutes claims made by animal rights activists, reveals what it says are hidden agendas of animal rights groups, and protects the rights of Americans to eat meat, drink milk, wear fur, and visit zoos.

The Animal's Voice (www.animalsvoice.com). The Animal's Voice is an online resource for animal defenders. It includes investigative reports, editorials, and news about animal rights activism.

Religious Thought About Animals (http://online.sfsu.edu/~rone/ Religion/religionanimals.html). This Web site, compiled by a religious studies professor, includes articles and links discussing animal rights and how animals are treated and viewed in various religious traditions.

Index

Picture Credits

Cover: © Michael Prince/CORBIS
Maury Aaseng, 35, 86, 92, 98
AFP/Getty Images, 41, 59
AP/Wide World Photos, 12, 49, 50, 66, 97, 104, 108
© Bettmann/CORBIS, 81
© Claro Cortes IV/Reuters/CORBIS, 52
© Rick Friedman/CORBIS, 28
Getty Images, 18, 43, 73, 76, 93
Tim Graham/Getty Images, 11
© Martin Harvey/CORBIS, 14
© Ali Jarekji/Reuters/CORBIS, 34
© Karen Kasmauski/CORBIS, 62
© Andrew Lichenstein/CORBIS, 68
© Robert Maass/CORBIS, 85
David McNew/Getty Images, 17
© Jack Naegelen/Reuters/CORBIS, 24
National Geographic/Getty Images, 42
People for the Ethical Treatment of Animals (PETA), 55, 56
© Steve Prezant/CORBIS, 29
© Carl & Ann Purcell/CORBIS, 23
Boris Reossler/DPA/Landov, 88
© Reuters/CORBIS, 31, 47, 65
© *Time* Magazine/Handout/Reuters/CORBIS, 102
Pierre Verdy/AFP/Getty Images, 10
© Haruyoshi Yamaguchi/CORBIS, 36

About the Editor

William Dudley received his BA degree from Beloit College in Wisconsin, where he majored in English composition and wrote for the school newspaper and literary journal. He has since written and published op-ed pieces, travel articles, and other pieces of writing. He has edited dozens of books on history and social issues for Greenhaven Press at Thomson/Gale.